P9-CMA-506

Springer Series on Medical Education

SERIES EDITOR: Steven Jonas, M.D.

Robert Henry Ross, PhD, is a sociologist of higher education and the professions who has studied at Yale University (MA, PhD, Sociology), Harvard University (EdM, Education), Dartmouth College (BA, Philosophy), and Union Theological Seminary (New York City). Dr. Ross has held Fulbright-Hays and Social Science Research Council grants and conducted field research in the United States, Canada, Great Britain, and Italy. His current interests include health professions education and practice and health policy research trends.

Dr. Ross has taught at the Harvard School of Public Health and at Wellesley, Harvard, and Yale Colleges. Now a research associate at the Health Institute of the New England Medical Center, Tufts University, he was formerly a research associate with the Dean's Office at the Harvard School of Public Health and a visiting fellow at the New England Resource Center for Higher Education at the University of Massachusetts, Boston.

Harvey V. Fineberg, MD, PhD, is Dean of the Harvard School of Public Health. He is a graduate of Harvard College, Harvard Medical School, and Harvard's John F. Kennedy School of Government. Prior to his appointment as dean in 1984, he was a professor in health policy and management at the School of Public Health.

Since the 1970s, Dean Fineberg has been a leading figure in the health policy field. As a member of the Public Health Council of Massachusetts from 1976–1979, he participated in decision-making matters of hospital investment and health policy. From 1982 to 1985 he served as chairman of the Health Care Technology Study Section of the National Center for Health Services Research.

His past research has focused on several areas of health policy, including the process of policy development and implementation, assessment of medical technology, and dissemination of medical innovations. He helped found and has served as president of the Society for Medical Decision Making and has also served as a consultant to the World Health Organization. As a member of the Institute of Medicine, he has served on numerous panels dealing with topics of health policy, ranging from AIDS to vaccines to new medical technology.

Springer Series on Medical Education

Innovators IN Physician Education

The Process and Pattern of Reform in North American Medical Schools

Robert H. Ross, PhD

Harvey V. Fineberg, MD, PhD

SPRINGER PUBLISHING COMPANY

Springer Publishing Company, Inc.
536 Broadway
New York, NY 10012-3955

Cover design by Tom Yabut
Production Editor: Pamela Lankas

96 97 98 99 00 / 5 4 3 2 1

Library of Congress Cataloging-in-Publication Data

Ross, Robert H., Ph.D.
   Innovators in physician education : the process and pattern of
reform in North American medical schools / Robert H. Ross,
Harvey V. Fineberg.
      p.   cm. — (Springer series on medical education : 1995)
   Includes bibliographical references and index.
   ISBN 0-8261-9200-9
   1. Medical colleges—United States—Curricula—Case studies.
2. Educational change—United States—Case studies.   3. Medical
colleges—Canada—Curricula—Case studies.   4. Educational change—
Canada—Case studies.   I. Fineberg, Harvey V.   II. Title.
III. Series.
   ([DNLM: 1. Education, Medical—trends—Canada.   2. Education,
Medical—trends—United States.   3. Schools, Medical—Canada.
4. Schools, Medical—United States.   W 18 F4951 1996 / W1 SP685SE
1995 1996]
R743.F54   1996
610'.71'173—dc20
DNLM/DLC
for Library of Congress   95-40280
                                                                              CIP

Printed in the United States of America

Contents

Acknowledgments

The authors gratefully acknowledge 2 years' research support provided by the Robert Wood Johnson Foundation. We also thank Gordon Moore, MD, Director of Teaching Programs at the Harvard Community Health Plan, who provided good counsel and useful information at an early point in the research. At the Harvard School of Public Health, work could not have proceeded without the administrative and editorial contributions of Bernita L. Anderson, special assistant to the dean; the logistical and record-keeping services of Sarah K. Wood, senior administrative assistant to the dean; and the dean's office secretarial support of Renée L. Graham and Laura H. Hercod. Mr. Carl Morris, Harvard Medical School student, helped conduct the literature search, and Ms. Rosie Lynn and Mr. Mack Rhinelander turned tape recordings and interview field notes into document files.

The survey instrument that guided these interviews drew on an earlier questionnaire that Dr. Ross had co-designed in 1989–1990 while he was a research associate at the New England Resource Center for Higher Education, University of Massachusetts, Boston, with colleagues Zelda Gamson, PhD, Director, and Fellows Sandra Kanter, PhD, and Howard London, PhD.

The authors sincerely thank the many interviewees, who were promised anonymity, at each of 10 subject schools who gave an hour or more of their time in the midst of busy schedules. For permitting ten site visits in the first place, we are grateful to the deans, W. Douglas Skelton, MD, Christian L. Gulbrandsen, MD, Leonard M. Napolitano, PhD, David M. Brown, MD, Neil S. Cherniack, MD, Andrew G. Wallace, MD,

Daniel C. Tosteson, MD, Joseph B. Martin, MD, PhD, John Bienenstock, MD, and Michael A. Bureau, MD. For assistance in arranging our visits, we likewise thank Robert J. Moon, PhD at Mercer; S. Scott Obenshain, MD and Ms. Donna Baker at New Mexico; Satoru Izutsu, PhD and Ms. Gayle Gilbert at Hawaii; Robert J. McCollister, MD and Ms. Annette Roth Boorsma at Minnesota; David P. Stevens, MD, Ms. Lois Kaye, and Ms. Beth Shapiro at Case Western Reserve; William J. Culp, PhD and Ms. Judy Emery at Dartmouth; Daniel D. Federman, MD and Ms. Anne Hallward at Harvard; Emily Osborn, MD, MPH, Ms. Kathleen Healy, and Ms. Helen Hong at UCSF; Mr. Kevin Smith at McMaster; and Jacques Des Marchais, MD at Sherbrooke. Finally, we gratefully acknowledge the MD students who shared their thoughts with us, including R. Mosley, B. Berard, C. Vaughn, and J. Roberts at Mercer; K. Goodluck, K. Bordenave, and D. Buckley at New Mexico; H. Lee, S. Ayabe, B. Ueno, and K. Mack at Hawaii; K. Miller, R. Baker, K. Wyche, H. Boyer, A. Vainio, K. Abtin, P. Stachowicz, J. Smith, and D. Hartsuch at Minnesota; A. Picken, R. Zimmerman, A. Campbell, M. Stewart, and S. Lord at Case Western Reserve; E. Chapman, S. Weiner, and D. Reineke at Dartmouth; D. Hoffer, A. Jha, A. Hallward, J. MacDonald, R. Emani, and E. Gantt at Harvard; J. Morena, A. Lee, L. Burkholder, D. Li, and M. Pretzer at UCSF; K. Kontio, B. Thorogood, S. Shaver, and P. Labreque at McMaster; M. De Bujanda, A. Dupras, T. Tremblay, C. Marriott, and J.A. Bourque at Sherbrooke.

Preface

The purpose of this volume is to inform continuing efforts to improve general professional medical education in the U.S. and Canada. It is not to advocate any one method. If reform theory circulates widely nowadays, reform practice remains local, closely conditioned in design and implementation by ground-level circumstances, less a received program than an adaptive process a learning from experience.

Text and commentary are interwoven here, and the truth is in the details. The text is primary, narration that could only be supplied by the actors themselves. Commentary is secondary, the authors' interpretation that could be supplied as well by other thoughtful readers. Text comes from interviews conducted with administrators, faculty, and students at ten North American medical schools from October 1991 through February 1992. Like the change process it recounts, the text is iterative, a running narrative in eight chapters concerning the context (part 1), process (part 2), and subjects (part 3) of curriculum and related change at each of ten cases studied. Though each case is unique, all ten, having selected from an extended family of current-cycle reform ideas, bear certain resemblances.

Throughout this volume, text is presented in indented passages following each paragraph of commentary. The lead passage under each new paragraph, and any subsequent passage attributable to a respondent other than the immediately preceding one, is always indicated by a bullet (•). The method throughout is plainly ethnographic. Text necessarily and intentionally expresses the points of view of respondents.

Several phrases in this volume are routinely cut short, for convenience, into single words. First, "innovator" and "innovation" are rarely accompanied by "educational," though it is always implied. Second, "Harvard," for example, is rarely accompanied by "medical school," let alone "medical school MD program," though it is likewise implied. Third, the medical school at the University of California, San Francisco is always rendered "UCSF." Bracketed material in text beginning with "I:" indicates an interviewer question or comment, that without, a condensation of material.

By painstaking transcription of interview and field notes, we have sought faithfully to convey respondents' views. We solicited reviews for accuracy and fairness of pertinent text from designated officers at each participating school and adapted text accordingly. For remaining inaccuracies, of person or place names for example, as indeed for our selection and interpretation of text, we bear full responsibility and welcome correction or comment.

Introduction

If the number of recent articles, reports, and monographs[1] devoted to the subject is any indication, North American medical education is in considerable ferment today. In fact, as Figure I.1 indicates, this ferment arrives at the high point of a reform cycle, the century's third after Flexner's science-centered and Western Reserve's organ-centered reforms.[2] The present cycle, as we see it, begins with the 1960s' reassessment of strictly biomedical science-based medical education;[3] continues to build through the 1970s in variations of problem-based, patient-centered, community-oriented, primary care-focused programs at schools like McMaster and New Mexico;[4] reaches full conceptualization in the 1984 *GPEP Report*;[5] and grows into the 1980s' and early 1990s' widespread reconsideration and reconfiguration of educational practice, which this book seeks to exemplify.

Physicians for the Twenty-First Century, Report of the Panel on the General Professional Education of the Physician and College Preparation for Medicine, known colloquially as the *GPEP Report* (after the initials contained in its subtitle), was written by a distinguished panel of medical educators convened in the early 1980s by the Association of American Medical Colleges. The major reassessment of the structure and functioning of predoctoral medical education in the present period, it is divided into five major conclusions—covering the purposes of general professional medical education, premedical baccalaureate education, learning skills in medical school, clinical medical education, and medical faculty involvement—each divided into a series of specific recommendations. In the decade since the *GPEP Report* most of the 126 U.S. and 16 Canadian medical schools have undertaken general professional education reform

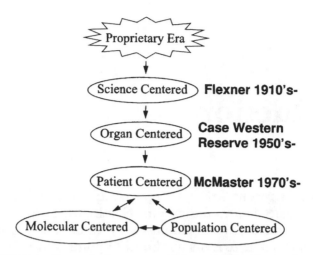

FIGURE I.1. Twentieth-century reform in medical education.

of greater or lesser scope. By the mid-1990s, moreover, U.S. and Canadian medical schools alike know full well that impending financial and organizational restructuring of health care systems will require further hand-in-glove adaptations of medical education.

FORCES FOR CHANGE

Looking back,[6] it is the intense development and differentiation of biomedical science and technology over the past quarter century that has driven the equally intense differentiation of medical education and medical practice. Throughout the 1970s and 1980s, increasingly lengthy training for a burgeoning number of specialties became the norm in medical education, as generalists nearly became an endangered species. Now, despite evidence that there are still too many of the former and too few of the latter relative to actual needs, the trend persists into the 1990s, even as remedies are sought to reverse it.[7]

A combination of factors—academic, professional, political, and social—appears to have created the problem. Faculties of medicine, built up from increasingly differentiated discipline-based basic and clinical science departments, have readily configured medical education in their own subdisciplinary image for purposes of managing academic careers and procuring institutional resources. So doing, they have inadvertently blocked consideration of which other poles—developing teaching and research across disciplines, more student-centered learning, community service, for example—the medical education tent might also be pitched on. Societies of practitioners, built up in turn from increasingly differentiated bodies of scientific–technical expertise, have likewise configured medical practice in their own subspecialist image for purposes of controlling access to advanced practice and securing professional standards. And they, in turn, have inadvertently blocked consideration of which other poles—integrating medical science and technology across specialties, more patient- and community-centered practice, for example—the medical practice tent might also be pitched on.

For their part, until recently, state and federal legislators and executives have been slow to comprehend and promote alternatives to subspecialty medical practice and the medical insurance industry that underwrites it. Even now, "health care policy" remains suspect in many political circles, as a routine reading of the nation's editorial pages will confirm. Organized sectors in society—business, labor, retirees, for example—have also, until recently, promoted high-tech, tertiary care, specialist medicine over more integrated primary-to-tertiary health care. Unorganized populations with no voice and little access to services of any sort, the working poor and the transient especially, have not been heard, of course. Popular beliefs, reinforced by the experts, have long served to legitimate the myth of expertise and to obscure the logic and possibility of primary and preventive health care.

Yet, undeniably, pressure for change has mounted in recent years. Through the 1980s, discontent with economic stagnation, too much government borrowing, and huge federal deficits fueled an electoral realignment that, by the early 1990s, ushered a president into office pledged in the medical arena to creating more accessible, affordable health care. Over the same time period, health maintenance organizations and other managed care systems, state by state, were increasing demand for and elevating the status of generalists in the fields of internal medicine, family practice, obstetrics–gynecology, and pediatrics.

A number of forces—here, too, academic, professional, political, and social—have fostered demands for change. In the last quarter century, internal challenges to the strictly biomedical model of medical education have been manifest in medical school efforts—here administration-driven, there faculty-led, often piecemeal, sometimes sweeping—to reconfigure mission, curriculum, teaching, research, even admissions. Comparable challenges to the strictly specialist model of medical practice have likewise been manifest in the efforts of physicians in primary and family care fields to elevate general practice to specialty status per se.[8]

The orientation of a growing number of politicians, at both the federal and state level, to medical services has also shifted markedly in recent years from being deferential to the medical establishment to a more activist, problem-solving, delivery-oriented approach. The shift has been prompted not only by public outcry for greater access and affordability but also by the pronouncements of a growing number of medical educators and practitioners themselves. Calls are increasingly heard at the public and professional levels for more integrated health care delivery, community and population medicine, health promotion and disease prevention efforts, even provision for excluded populations. New norms such as the "informed patient," "joint decision-making," and "information-sharing" likewise gained credence through the 1980s, corresponding to a downturn of popular belief in an omniscient, disinterested medical profession.

THE INNOVATORS

With most North American medical schools in recent years considering and initiating efforts to adapt educational practice to such calls for change, it seemed an opportune moment to go out among the innovators of some duration, to assess the nature and scope of their reform efforts, and to present our findings to the entire community. We defined as innovators those schools that had made serious efforts to design and implement significant reform before the start of the present decade, ones therefore that would have an established record by the time we commenced field work in the fall of 1992.[9]

So defining the universe served several purposes. It provided a pool of possible cases that numbered more than the relatively few long-standing innovators, ones whose reform efforts often reached back into the 1970s, but fewer than the very many that by 1990 were actively reconsidering how they should instruct medical students. It also established the first of three institutional characteristics that we thought might affect the manner in which schools innovate, what we call their reform "posture" in the current reform cycle, namely, earlier or later innovator status.

We made 1980 the cutoff year between earlier and later innovators so that the former might have worked with less and the latter with more benefit of hindsight, blueprint, or received record. We wondered whether later innovators like UCSF or Hawaii might not innovate more boldly, because they were better informed, than earlier innovators like McMaster or New Mexico. Similarly, we wondered whether earlier reform-cycle innovators like Case Western or Minnesota[10] might not define themselves as "having innovated" so much so that they were less receptive, or more selectively receptive, to current-cycle GPEP-style ideas about change. We reasoned that findings from the study might be more relevant to our intended audience, the entire medical education community, if as many later as earlier innovators were included among cases studied. We thought that the many noninnovators, schools that by 1990–1991 had yet, by our definition, to make a serious effort at significant reform might have more to learn from the later innovators, which they more resemble in received record and reform timing

The second characteristic that we thought might affect a school's reform posture is its juridical status, namely whether it is public or private. Public schools may be more and private schools less mission-constrained, we thought, as a result of being more and less tethered, respectively, to public legislatures. Public schools may draw less and private schools more on a nationwide applicant pool as a result of being more and less bound, respectively, to capitation and other state grants, which in some states may even affect the quality of applicant pools. Practical state legislators, for their part, may define MD program graduates, more than residents and fellows, as the first order of business. For these reasons, we thought, the public schools might be prone to innovate less. It occurred to us too, however, that private schools are more tuition-dependent than public schools, thus more expensive, which may in its own way winnow applicant pools. In contrast to the better public schools that may return each year to stable sources of fixed revenue, the less-endowed private schools can be more dependent on variable funding, which in turn may diminish their propensity to innovate. On balance, we speculated that the private schools might be more and the public schools less innovative.

Third, we thought that whether a school was older or younger with respect to founding date might affect its reform posture and, for this, we made 1960 the cutoff year. We were not alone in thinking that how "well-founded" a school feels itself might affect its receptivity to innovation.

> Change is possible but it seems to come from either the brand "new" schools which start with pencil and paper or from the great "old" schools which may take a giant leap forward every couple of generations. (Ebert & Ginzberg, 1988, p. 63)

In this sense schools more remotely and more recently established may be better poised to experiment.

In this manner, then, we arrived at the first three columns of Table I.1.[11] We arrived at the fourth column by accessing files, under strict confidentiality, of 67 U.S. schools' applications to a leading foundation's recent initiative to encourage innovation in predoctoral medical education. The application for this program required schools to detail their records in curricular and administrative reform and to outline any such future intentions. We closely read these sections of each application and so selected 30 of the 32 schools listed in Table I.1 judged to have most extensively innovated.[12] Reviewing the literature, we also kept a sharp eye for any innovator that might not have applied to the above program and, in this way, located one very strong case and found another that had in fact applied to the program

TABLE I.1 A Typology of Medical Education Innovators

Sector public/private	Founded (4 yr) 1960 cutoff	Innovator 1980 cutoff	Schools (N = 32)
Public	Older	Earlier	Minnesota, Ohio State
"	"	Later	Illinois, Nebraska, Oregon, UCLA, UCSF, UNC-Chapel Hill
"	Younger	Earlier	Michigan State, Missouri-KC, New Mexico, S. Illinois
"	"	Later	Hawaii, Kentucky, N. Dakota, S. Dakota W. Virginia
Private	Older	Earlier	Case Western, Johns Hopkins
"	"	Later	Bowman-Gray, Chicago, Columbia, Cornell, Harvard, Rochester, Stanford, Tufts, Yale
"	Younger	Earlier	Brown, Mercer
"	"	Later	Dartmouth, Rush

but whose application left us with an incomplete impression of reform efforts.

With 32 cases spread among eight groups, we devised a method to choose two leading candidates from each of the four cells that contained more than two schools.[13] Our final selection, one case from each of eight pairs, was made with an eye to the geographic and urban/rural distribution of cases and so as to include among earlier innovators two from the previous 1950s–1960s reform cycle. In this way we produced the following list of U.S. schools.

> public, older, earlier innovator: **University of Minnesota**
> public, older, later innovator: **University of California, San Francisco**
> public, younger, earlier innovator: **University of New Mexico**
> public, younger, later innovator: **University of Hawaii**
> private, older, earlier innovator: **Case Western Reserve University**
> private, older, later innovator: **Harvard University**
> private, younger, earlier innovator: **Mercer University**
> private, younger, later innovator: **Dartmouth College**

For Canada, we chose a leading innovator on each side of that country's Anglophone-Francophone division, respectively, **McMaster University** and the **University of Sherbrooke.** To the deans of these medical schools we then wrote letters explaining the purpose of our research and inviting them to participate in the study. Happily, each accepted the offer.[14]

The 10 medical schools in our study are as diverse institutionally as they are dispersed geographically (see Figure I.2). In the beginning (of the present reform cycle) were New Mexico, in Albuquerque, and McMaster, in Hamilton, Ontario. Both were founded in the upbeat 1960s and both have since pioneered waves of small-group, problem-based, primary-care-oriented, population-based medical education, McMaster across-the-board, New Mexico down one track.

Mercer, in Macon, Georgia, is the youngest fully accredited and one of the smallest U.S. medical schools. Of the 10 it has the most distinct mission, to train physicians for the state's ru-

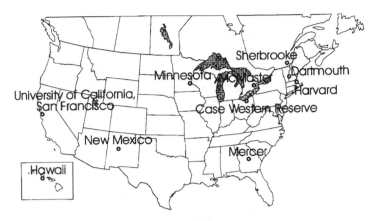

FIGURE I.2 Participating medical schools.

ral and underserved populations. Sherbrooke, in Quebec, like Mercer the youngest and smallest in its own province, also, and for quite comparable strategic reasons, created an entirely problem-based curriculum in the 1980s, which is now fully operational. Like Sherbrooke, though even more recently, Hawaii, in Honolulu, converted across-the-board from traditional lecture-lab to problem-based, small-group instruction. Like New Mexico, Hawaii is the sole medical school in its state, however, and has benefited accordingly from the same greater latitude to experiment.

Of two previous-cycle innovators in the study, Minnesota so epitomizes the big medical school ensconced in a far-flung, research-oriented academic medical center that innovation efforts in teaching and learning are, nearly by necessity, generated individually on location rather than planned collectively from central offices. Case Western Reserve, in turn, in Cleveland, Ohio, maintains the time-honored tradition of admitting unusual and unusually talented students and of giving them great leeway in their studies, even as the school aspires to become a major force in medical research in the 1990s.

Harvard, in Boston, Massachusetts, is as heterodox a medical school as Dartmouth, in Hanover, New Hampshire, has been orthodox. At Harvard, the dean-inspired New Pathway experiment ran well enough through the 1980s, alongside the more

traditional curriculum and within an otherwise medical-bio-re-
search-and-technology-driven environment, to see its tutorial
format and doctor–patient focus integrated across the entire
predoctoral program by the 1990s. Dartmouth, for most of the
century a 2-year biomedical sciences program, switched to the
4-year curriculum in the 1970s. Since attracting a few key faculty and administrators in the 1980s and completing a major
new academic medical center complex in the early 1990s, Dartmouth is now reconfiguring, without much tranquility, its
rather traditional curriculum.

The University of California at San Francisco (UCSF) is
Harvard's public counterpart in faculty research and student
caliber, but it differs in graduating fully half of its recent MD
classes with a variety of primary-care orientations. Confined on
top of Parnassus hill, UCSF knows that its ongoing excellence
will depend on solving its space constraint problem.

CHANGE PROCESS

How then do present-day medical schools innovate? How do they
go about changing educational programs? Are schools predis-
posed to change differently? How does change get going? unfold? resolve? Does the process differ among schools, and, if so,
why? These, the pivotal questions of this volume, should be clarified in several important respects before we seek to answer
them in the eight chapters that follow.

First, we think of change in general professional medical
education as a *process*, an eventful sequence, a play in several
acts.[15] How each act plays out is consequential for the next and
thus for the entire production. Three acts—impetus, design, implementation—may be identified in the change process that interests us. We sought answers, reported in part 2, to four broad
questions at each of ten subject schools:

- Impetus: Why did people want to change the medical education program?
- Design: Who designed the changes and how did they go
  about it?

- Implementation: How was the new program implemented and what changes were subsequently made?
- Lessons: What was learned over the process concerning how and how not to innovate?

Second, we think of change as a process in *context*, context that includes a school's mission, its particular problems, and the morale of its faculty. Context may vary, then, by how the mission is defined, by how fundamental its problems are, and by how attached faculty members are to the school. In part 1, we examine how the change process that interests us is contextualized by:

- School mission: Schools may be more mission-comprehensive (teaching, research, service) or mission-distinct (primarily teaching, service).
- Major problems: Schools may have problems that are more structural (actual survival, for example) or more situational (an increasingly competitive health care environment, for example).
- Faculty morale: Schools may have more or less institutionally identified and attached faculty, thus better or worse schoolwide morale and inclination to get involved in change.

Third, we think of change as a process that is *patterned* according to change sponsorship, or who engenders it, to change scope, or what it seeks to alter, and to the change consequences, or how well it succeeds. In part 2, we will also examine how the change process that interests us is patterned by:

- Sponsorship: Change may be more administration-led (top–down) or faculty-driven (bottom–up), or it may be co-sponsored.
- Scope: Change may be more wholesale (across-the-board) or within-bounds ("across a row" or "down a column").[16]
- Consequence: Change may be more institution-or person-embodied, thus more or less lasting in its effects.

Finally, we think that the change process itself is probably conditioned by schools' defining *institutional characteristics—*

public-private, older-younger, earlier-later innovator status—by which we stratified the universe from which we drew the sample for our study. Ways in which these characteristics may influence change will be examined throughout parts 1 and 2 and in the conclusion of the report.

In part 3, finally, we listen closely, school by school, to what the students—those who ultimately benefit or not from innovation—appreciate most and least about their medical education to date and what they imagine, once in their practices, they will appreciate most and least in retrospect. From these evaluations we draw several conclusions concerning how students' evaluations of their educational experience may differ according to the type of innovation that their schools have undertaken.

We have written this volume with the idea that as change is initiated, designed, and implemented, important features emerge as to who prompts the change, how broad a change is intended, and what outcome is achieved, according to how mission-comprehensive or mission-distinct, problem-structural or problem-situational, and faculty-attached or faculty-detached schools are, and according to their public–private, older–younger, and earlier–later innovator status (Figure I.3). It will suit our purpose if these 10, diverse reform experiences inform further innovation efforts. The utility of the study and the patterns it reveals depends on whether and how it facilitates discussion among current cycle reform in yay-, nay-, and may-sayers alike concerning the limits of the possible in medical education. We hope that it sheds light on a sometimes dimly lit debate.

NOTES

1. For a bibliography, 1976–1990, that lists some 392 articles under headings such as school funding and governance, curriculum development, problem-based learning, admissions, clinical skills assessment, and faculty development, see M. Teresa Nigro and Rebekah J. Lynn, *Reading in medical education: Sources of innovative ideas,* second edition, Assessing Change in Medical Education-The Road to Implementation (ACME-TRI) Project. For an update since 1990, see entries dated 1991 and following in the references to this volume.

2. See Abraham Flexner, *Medical education in the United States and*

Change Context

School mission
Major problems
Faculty morale

School Characteristics

Public-private
Older-younger
Earlier-later innovator

Change Process and Pattern

Impetus and sponsorship
Design and scope
Implementation and consequences

FIGURE I.3 Dimensions of change in medical schools.

Canada, and Greer Williams, *Western Reserve's experiment in medical education and its outcome.*

    3. See chapters by Hughes and Thorne in Everett C. Hughes et al., *Education for the professions of medicine, law, theology, and social welfare.*

    4. For McMaster, see William B. Spaulding, in collaboration with Janet Cochran, *Revitalizing medical education: McMaster medical school, the early years 1965–1974;* for New Mexico, Arthur Kaufman (Ed.), *Implementing problem-based medical education: Lessons from successful innovations,* Arthur Kaufman et al., "The New Mexico experiment: Educational innovation and institutional change," and Arthur Kaufman, "Rurally based education: Confronting social forces underlying ill health."

    5. The panel's recommendations are summarized in Appendix 2, *The GPEP Report,* this volume.

    6. The contents of this and the remaining five paragraphs condense those presented in Appendix 1: Voices for Change, itself a 15-part synthesis of Robert H. Ebert and Eli Ginzberg's "The reform of medical education," David S. Greer's "Altering the mission of the academic health center: Can medical schools really change?," Charles E. Odegaard's *Dear doctor: A personal letter to a physician,* Kerr White's *The task of medicine: dialogue at Wickenden,* and *The Pew Health Professions Commission's Healthy America: Practitioners for 2005, an agenda for action for U.S. health professional schools.*

    7. The specialist–generalist debate took center stage by the early 1990s. See Association of American Medical Colleges, "AAMC policy on the

generalist physician"; B. Barzansky et al., "A view of medical practice in 2020 and its implications for medical school admission"; W.T. Butler, "Academic medicine's season of accountability and social responsibility"; R.G. Christiansen et al., "A proposal for a combined family practice-internal medicine residency"; J.M. Colwill, "Education for the primary physician: A time for reconsideration?"; J.R. Evans, "The 'health of the public' approach to medical education"; J.P. Geyman, "Training primary care physicians for the 21st century"; M.R. Greenlick, "Educating physicians for population-based clinical practice"; J.S. Jonas et al., "Educational programs in US medical schools"; D.G. Kassebaum et al., "The declining interest of medical school graduates in generalist specialties: Students' abandonment of earlier inclinations"; J.L. Murray et al., "A national, interdisciplinary consortium of primary care organizations to promote the education of generalist physicians"; H.K. Rabinowitz, "Evaluation of a selective medical school admissions policy to increase the number of family physicians in rural and under-served areas"; S.A. Schroeder, "Training an appropriate mix of physicians to meet the nation's needs"; A.H. Strelnick et al., "Graduate primary care training: A collaborative alternative for family practice, internal medicine, and pediatrics"; A.R. Tarlov, "The coming influence of a social sciences perspective on medical education"; J.E. Verby et al., "Changing the medical school curriculum to improve patient access to primary care"; M.E. Whitcome et al., "Comparing the characteristics of schools that produce high percentages and low percentages of primary care physicians."

8. For a sampling of such challenges, recorded in the 1980s, see the five essays included in Charles Odegaard's *Dear doctor,* including George L. Engel, "How much longer must medicine's science be bound by a seventeenth century world view?"; Michael A. Schwartz and Osborn P. Wiggins, "Scientific and humanistic medicine: A theory of clinical methods"; G. Gayle Stephens, "Reflections of a post-Flexnerian physician"; Leon Eisenberg, "Science in medicine: Too much or too little or too limited in scope?"; and Ian R. McWhinney, "Through clinical methods to a more humanistic medicine."

9. We measured the extent of reform by the correspondence of a school's innovation effort to the range of recommendations contained in Appendix 2, *The GPEP Report,* this volume. Our way of identifying innovative cases, in its results, resembles that adopted by Charles Friedman et al., in "Charting the winds of change: Evaluating innovative medical curricula."

10. See Greer Williams, *Western Reserve's experiment in medical education and its outcome,* and J.E. Verby, "The Minnesota rural physician associate program for medical students."

11. We did not think to stratify the universe with a fourth characteristic—size, an indicator of organizational complexity—which, we will see, appears to affect both the context and pattern of innovation among schools. For comparison, figures for subject schools' 1991–1992 first-year class entrants [of which out-of-state entrants] followed by tuition and fees charged [nonresident tuition, if public] are as follow: **Mercer,** 47 [0], $14,714 + $702; **Hawaii,** 56

[3], $5,050 + $87 [$15,830]; **New Mexico** 73 [7], $3,300 + $32 [$9,300]; **Minnesota** 180 [49], $8,868 + $354 [$17,736]; **Case Western Reserve,** 138 [52], $18,200 + $250; **Dartmouth** 88 [81], $21,065 + $960; **Harvard** 165 [151], $19,110 + $1,542; **UCSF** 141 [34], None + $2,952 [$7,698]; **McMaster** 100 [13], $3,375 + $315 [$14,430]; **Sherbrooke** 102 [14], $1,967 + $1,500 [$10,440]. Numbers for comparison to the latter two cases are for **Toronto** 251 [25], $2,251 + $297 [$10,877] and **Montreal** 174 [10], $1,594 + $150 [$6,960]. See Association of American Medical Colleges, *Medical school admission requirements, 1993–94, United States and Canada,* 43rd edition. In 1992 a U.S. dollar equalled approximately $1.25 Canadian.

12. Employing the foundation's applicant pool as a self-defined set of innovators among all 126 U.S. medical schools, we made two defensible assumptions: first, that actual innovators would almost certainly be found among applicants to a high-profile initiative in support of medical education innovation, especially considering how difficult funds for such purposes are to come by internally; second, that applying to the program, each applicant would be roughly equally motivated to set out what of significance it had actually implemented to date in the reform arena.

13. We analyzed 31 foundation applications plus one journal article detailing the 32nd case according to mention or not of specific GPEP-type innovations. For comparability, we standardized scores so obtained by dividing the total number of innovations in each case by two constants, based, respectively, on a comprehensive and a select list of such innovations. Comparing proportions so derived, we chose the two cases in each of these four groups that appeared to have the most extensive reform records.

14. We asked for a 2-or 3-day site visit, 12 or more interviewees, and 75-minute interview sessions. We asked to interview top administrators, key department heads, representative preclinical and clinical and senior and junior faculty, and a selection of students. We shared the interview schedules employed by the study—the "perceptions" and "design-implementation" questionnaires—ahead of time. The present volume is based on responses only to the "design-implementation" questionnaire.

15. For a study methodologically similar to our own, one that focuses on innovation process, see the four-school case study of curriculum reform by Margaret Bussigel et al., "Goal coupling and innovation in medical schools." For a dissimilar study, one that proposes a useful typology of innovation contents, see R.M. Harden et al., "Educational strategies in curriculum development: The SPICES model."

16. Readers may readily understand the concepts "wholesale" versus "within-bounds" change, as we intend them, by visualizing or referring to the program and curriculum tables common to medical school catalogues. In these, the rows often stand for successive years in a program, whereas the columns describe distinct programs, tracks, or pathways that may be followed through those years. Thus innovating "across a row," "across several rows," or "down a column" could mean, respectively, for example, bringing third-year

clinical material into second-year pathophysiology, joining elements of first-
and second-year courses in a new first-year combination, or creating a whole
new primary-care curriculum track. "Within-bounds" change by definition
cannot be "across-the-board" in that part or all of an old program remains in-
tact.

P_{ART} 1

Innovation Context

To introduce 10 schools in their own words and to reveal the context in which their various current-cycle innovation efforts have taken place, in part I we shall compare and contrast characteristics of school missions, major problems, and faculty morale. We will also examine whether certain institutional characteristics—schools' public or private, older or younger, earlier or later innovator status, also their size or institutional complexity—predispose them to change differently. Analytically and empirically these defining characteristics give warp to the weave of change context. Statements of school mission, we shall see, contrast with those of major problems in the way that the "might be" stands to the "actually is." Reports of faculty morale, like the judgments of students presented in part 3, will disclose in turn how innovation has been experienced at ground level, school by school.

In chapter 1, we will see that institution size does affect mission among the 10 schools that we have studied. Save Dartmouth, the smaller schools—those with roughly 100 or fewer annual MD admissions, including Mercer, Hawaii, New Mexico, McMaster, and Sherbrooke—deviate notably from the comprehensive do-it-all teaching–research–service mission. Compared to the bigger schools, each has adopted a more distinct calling, for example, to meet a state's or province's needs for primary-care or generalist physicians.

Because these five schools or faculties are public (except Mercer, which is one-third state-supported) and founded since 1960, a more distinct mission may also be related to having been recently spawned by and remaining tethered to one juridical expression or another of the public interest. That four of five

1

of these schools began operations in the socially experimental 1960s likewise suggests the importance for mission of a school's founding ethos. The same five schools, moreover, and only these five among the 10, were founded on or subsequently adopted GPEP-style experimental curricula in some combination of problem-based and community-oriented instruction so characteristic of present cycle reform. But for New Mexico, which is now merging its traditional and experimental tracks, innovation went across-the-board as well.

The schools with a more comprehensive mission (Minnesota, Case Western Reserve, Harvard, UCSF, and Dartmouth) are, save the last, bigger, more complex, and more functionally diverse. Authority cannot be as readily concentrated in these sometimes sprawling, necessarily more decentralized, institutions. Here, mission serves not so much as a unifying ideology as an overarching definition of the situation that may accommodate the many bases that these schools want to cover.

These five are also the older schools. Dartmouth, the nation's fourth oldest medical school, preserves the ambience of its comprehensive research-driven peers. Change at the older schools may also be startlingly innovative, as in Case Western's and Minnesota's 1950s and 1960s efforts, respectively, in organ- and committee-based medical education and in centered rural physician training, as well as in Harvard's New Pathway of the 1980s. But it cannot be global, because so much of so many sorts of teaching, research, and service activity is already in place. Although three in five of these schools are private, independent, and free to pursue excellence as they see fit, the two publics have also excelled, building top-rate mission-comprehensive programs with strong, steady support from their state assemblies.

In chapter 2, we will see that school size, age, and public–private status affect major problems, as these are described by respondents, less than mission does. This may be due to the ubiquity of present-day revenue difficulties at medical schools. Nearly every school reportedly suffers a fiscal shortfall of one sort or another. The small private schools, Mercer and Dartmouth, underfund their teaching missions. Big older public schools Minnesota and UCSF and the private ones, Case Western Reserve and Harvard, have seen severe cutbacks in federal and state support for research and other functions. In Canada,

McMaster and Sherbrooke have faced severe provincial recessions that eroded one's commitment to its founding ideology and nearly closed the other. All describe an internal sea change from education to research and service revenue imperatives that detract from teaching functions. Only the smaller new public schools, Hawaii and New Mexico, both preoccupied now with whole-school curriculum changeovers, fail to register strong financial worries.

Chapter 3 will show that size does bear directly on faculty morale, however, inasmuch as school problems may be experienced personally. What happens schoolwide at smaller Mercer, Hawaii, New Mexico, Dartmouth, McMaster, and Sherbrooke resonates in a way that it cannot at larger Minnesota, Case Western Reserve, Harvard, and UCSF, where activities of every sort, including curriculum reform, are necessarily more contained. Smaller means that neither the institution nor faculty roles can be quite as functionally differentiated given how more people are more involved in more things and thus experience more of what happens schoolwide. Smaller schools are abuzz in a way that larger schools cannot be. The bigger the problem— from polarization and uncertainty in the face of change to financial instability, even to survival threats—the bigger the buzz and the more broadly faculty morale is affected, in rising to or falling from the challenge. At the larger schools, so many are so much more specialized and more independent of the institution that fewer schoolwide problems can be personally experienced. Cutbacks in research support affect researchers, competition for patients affects clinicians, tuition hikes affect students and teachers, and so forth. Only as dire a problem as UCSF's space constraint can put the whole place more than temporarily abuzz, and even then it may be considered the administration's problem.

If smaller schools require more diffuse faculty role performance than larger ones where research, teaching, and service roles are more differentiated, and if smaller ones too are more capable organizationally of innovating across-the-board, then it is also not surprising to find more reference at these schools, as we do in chapter 3, to faculty burnout, the anomie that comes from too much rather than too little engagement in schoolwide affairs.

CHAPTER 1

School Mission

Of the eight U.S. schools studied, it is the newer, smaller ones that have completely transformed the traditional lecture–lab curriculum, across-the-board at Mercer and Hawaii, and down an experimental track at New Mexico. It is these same schools that describe missions that deviate from the comprehensive education–research–service standard characteristic of the other five. To avow a mission that departs from the standard to which most American medical schools subscribe is by definition distinct.

The Mercer University School of Medicine is certainly unusual. The youngest fully accredited U.S. medical school, it is also an early innovator, founded fully problem-based in the late 1970s. Founders benefit from the received record and may even innovate blank-slate at first, but they must also soon enough define a niche that avoids head-on competition with the establishment, for Mercer represented by the Emory University School of Medicine and the Medical College of Georgia. Mercer's success has been based on a very distinct mission—to train physicians for rural and other underserved populations of Georgia in no less than six types of primary-care practice—in return for which the state underwrites a third of the private medical school's operating costs.

- [Our mission is to] turn out primary-care physicians for rural and medically underserved areas of Georgia. The mission began with family practice and grew. We would not have been LCME [Liaison Committee on Medical Education] accredited as only a family-practice school. This is why [the dean] has been so adamant. To him, the school has to do with general medicine, not on the one hand with research university medicine, nor on the other just with family practice. So we are not now going to expand into areas that we cannot support. We tell faculty in recruitment that there are limits. What we do, we are going to do well.

- [It is] to educate for primary care and other needed physicians to meet Georgia's health care needs in rural and other underserved areas. Therefore psychiatry was added by the Board of Governors as mission-compliant in 1986 or 1987. It is not primary care but it is mission-compliant. [Earlier] I went to the board to get the issue of general surgery clarified. I did not want to provoke a dispute at the national level over whether general surgery was or was not a primary-care field without at least board clarification. That is when the board declared that they only saw Mercer as a family practice school! So we had a big board meeting late in 1985 [where I called for] a vote over whether family practice was it as far as our mission was concerned. So the board voted to support the five areas: family practice, internal medicine, pediatrics, obstetrics–gynecology, and general surgery. The sixth, general psychiatry, was added later. Since then there have been occasional discussions within the board concerning other areas where a good case might be made for strong need in rural and underserved areas of Georgia, for example, emergency medicine or preventive medicine. But so far we have stayed within the six areas. [I: What is the key to remaining consistent with your mission?] Thirty percent of our students have state medical education scholarships of $6,000 annually. They must practice a year for every year they receive the scholarship in one of the five disciplines in communities acceptable to the state board. These are communities with populations under 15,000. For this one third of our students, if they do not do it, they owe the state three dollars for every one they were given. Other scholarships, for example, aid from a county, are tied to the same rules. [I: What is the proportion overall bound in this way?] About forty percent of our students. [I: So what is the key to remaining mission consistent at Mercer?] The biggest is how the school was formed. The next is how this curriculum was put together for specific reasons, highlighting primary care. And then the admissions process is very important. These three things—leadership, curriculum, admissions—must continually be put in front of us.

The John A. Burns School of Medicine at the University of Hawaii is fortunate in its geography. The state's only medical school, Hawaii, is less niche-constrained than Mercer. Leadership in such a case has an especially free hand to innovate, and at Hawaii it is being exercised as nowhere else. As a founding *ex nihilo* served Mercer, so a monopoly on in-state medical education served Hawaii, to invite top-down experiment, wholesale change. Hawaii's recent, sweeping innovation, like Mercer's, was across-the-board and mission-distinct.

- [Our mission is to] train primary care physicians. [I: Had we been speaking 8 to 10 years ago?] Same. [I: So the curriculum changes but the mission has stayed the same?] Yes. Whether the mission has been accomplished or not is a different question. [I: Was it more accomplished then or now?] I cannot say really on the basis of curriculum since our first problem-based learning class is just being graduated. We will have to see what they can do. My hunch is that there is not going to be that much of a change in graduates.
- The medical care system is in the sorry state that it is today largely because of physician training. Therefore medical schools are very greatly responsible for the state of medical care. Thus it is medical schools that should take the lead in changing how people behave in reforming the health care system. The medical schools need to identify their true customers. Ours are not our students but rather the public. The way I look at it, we are training the public's future employees. Therefore we must ask the public what they want their employees to do and not do, and train them accordingly. To do this we must connect the community not only to the health care system but also to medical education. That is what we are up to here. That is why we are forming community partnerships. We have three to date. We will have 11 when it is all done. It is a matter of money.

When the Kellogg Foundation came, they required that the community programs be financially self-sufficient after 5 years. I made the rounds of the legislature to ask that they show up at the breakfast with the Kellogg site visitors. They said to me, "Thank you for coming and telling us about this beforehand and thanks furthermore for not asking for any money!" I said, "Fine, but if this succeeds the community will come and knock down your doors for funding!" I myself will never ask the legislature for money. The sites will. That is why every one of the sites will be in a different legislative district. I want not only the network of health care partnerships but also a network of political connections to sustain them.

The University of New Mexico School of Medicine was an early pioneer. Unlike Mercer and Hawaii, therefore, it could benefit little from received record and thus adopted a more experimental within-bounds approach to innovation. A primary care curriculum track, parallel to but smaller than the traditional, was fashioned by the mid-1970s on the urging of a few clinical faculty, several of whom have worked side-by-side ever since. Now, as the experiment's proponents strive to forge a best-of-both curriculum of two long-separated tracks, they are opposed by basic scientists concerned that they will thus be curricularly disempowered. Mission is worded cautiously at New Mexico, perhaps to allow that the basic sciences not be slighted.

- To provide students with a variety of missions. To give students a broad enough background to build on for professional expertise in areas that are attractive to them. To fulfill both social and personal needs. The real problem that I see at this point in time is that the sciences relative to medicine are really getting at the central mechanisms that govern human biology. Thus, the real problem is to provide students with a framework in which therapies are going to be delivered in the next century.
- It is a mixed mission . . . to educate physicians for the state of New Mexico. This . . . means to be in tune with the needs the state has for primary-care physicians, but it also means to balance primary, secondary, and tertiary care in the

state. We still have to meet all these needs. The legislature really does not understand what they are paying for, because of the nature of the academic health center, which requires faculty and both patient care and laboratory work. A college of education, for example, does not run the schools but we do run the hospital and clinic and take care of patients. . . . There is no question that the institution has changed. For example, until 8 years ago, there was not even a department of anesthesiology. Now it is a big department. Also, the world view of certain chairs who came to this school early on to take on a dream has certainly changed significantly. It was a place that really did not have the money for that dream. In the early 1960s, the president of the University of New Mexico had no thought of us having a medical school here . . . but the legislature was finally convinced . . . largely to give state residents an opportunity to get a medical education and to provide more physicians for the state. So the founders went to Santa Fe, and got $100,000 to get the medical school started. Instead, they received $25,000 to hire a dean. It was the Kellogg Foundation grant that got things started actually.

The five remaining U.S. schools are bigger, organizationally more complex, less unified or, certainly, unifiable than Mercer, Hawaii, and New Mexico, and thus more representative of present-day medical schools. Because none of these more far flung institutions has or probably could have tried wholesale reform, within-bounds innovation efforts of greater and lesser magnitude have been undertaken.

The University of Minnesota School of Medicine, in doing everything and doing it well, is a prototype big public medical school. It innovated profoundly in the previous reform cycle, notably to train rural physicians, and may thus view itself now more as "having changed" than as "needing to change." Innovation at Minnesota in any case is bound to be at the margin, not from the center, incremental not wholesale, because the school, like the university, is so big, complex, and decentralized. Department- and discipline-based authority is nowhere stronger nor schoolwide education policy weaker than at big research-oriented medical schools like Minnesota, the sum, really, of their biomedical and clinical medicine departments. Leadership, selected from these ranks, focuses on research- and clinic revenue growth, keenly aware of mounting competition for patients. General professional medical education consumes only a tiny part of the budget and is left to a department-dominated curriculum committee. Mission is thus expressed in the broadest, most permissive terms possible.

- Education, research, patient care, and service. There are arrows up and back and forth among these. [I: And the relationship between undergraduate and graduate medical education, with respect to mission?] I regret that the current system separates graduate from undergraduate medical education in the way that it does. It is an artifact of the accreditation system. [I: What can you do about this?] You can reinforce the education component built into undergraduate through graduate medical education. You can reinforce the basic sciences and their relevance to medicine. You can inform clinical medicine more profoundly by its basic science foundations. You can use basic science content to help explain clinical diagnostics, treatment, and medication. [Five years from now,] the responsibility for graduate medical education oversight will be within the medical school, not within each department. It will be this oversight activity that is the springboard for getting more involved with the curricular side of things. We will organize graduate medical education committees schoolwide. [The competitive health care environment in Minnesota] made us realize that we have to compete in order to assure the patient input to the hospitals that we need. This in turn has brought about an internal change of behavior and policies among all the physicians in the university hospitals in relation to students, patients, referring physicians, and payers. Most health care economists would agree that Minnesota has one of the most highly competitive health care environments of any state in the nation.
- [Mission] is to accept the most academically competent group of students that we can . . . and to provide them the best possible medical education. Ten years ago, I would have confined my definition to Minnesota, but we liberal-

ized our admissions criteria recently and so 20% of our students are now non-Minnesotans. The dean's directives in this regard in the late 1980s were coincidental with the falling number of applicants of the period. We also had to reduce class size. In 1984 our class stood at 229, whereas in 1991 it came to 185. Keep in mind that we take 48 students from the 2–year program in Duluth.

The Case Western Reserve University School of Medicine is fretful. A previous reform-cycle innovator in 1950s committee-run, organ-systems-based medical education, Case Western Reserve still professes trademark commitment to general professional medical education, even as leadership pushes the school to compete and excel in the 1990s big biomedical science research environment. Some feel that the teaching mission has lost ground.

• The purpose of the medical education program [in the 1950s] according to the draft that we wrote in 1952 was simply to produce good doctors . . . "blast" physicians. Blast cells, of course, are those in bone marrow that differentiate into a wide variety of cell types. Thus we wanted our students to differentiate into a wide variety of specialty types. The corollary to this was that our students would participate in continuing education for the rest of their professional lives [and] that there should thus be a limit on the content of teaching to restrict the total mass of material imparted. We also insisted that, in patient care, our students pay attention to the individual as much as to the disease. When the curriculum was set up in the 1950s, it was divided into subject committees by organ systems. These were reorganized in phases after the year 1968. In the 1950s and 1960s, therefore, the subject committee chairs were the dominant figures in the medical school and the chairs altogether were supervised by a coordinator appointed for 3 to 5 years. I was first the chair of the kidney committee and then coordinator for 5 years. If you do that, you do so somewhat at the expense of your academic career, because you are interested in it. Many of these people approached their subjects and their teaching with real feeling. More recently, however, the economics of the school is said to be the dominant consideration. [I: What motivated them?] When people came back from World War II they felt that they could do anything. I served on a destroyer, for example. Second, people gave expression to an almost hidden pleasure in teaching in those days. You had to be a skilled scientist or physician certainly, but teaching then was not only respected but desirable. People recalled the bad parts of their own education and wanted to change this in their own teaching. It was a young faculty then and they had a voice. The Committee on Medical Education had a dozen subcommittees, and everyone had a say.

- The main part [of mission] is education. The school has always looked at itself as training "blast" physicians, but I am not sure that this is the correct mission. It may be that the mission of the school should be to train leaders of all sorts, including leaders in research, that the school should be more research oriented. Until now, the school has been primarily a bench-research-oriented school, but there are other forms of research, too, such as population based. Important to many faculty and students here, but not so much in my mind, is the perception of a service mission of the medical school.

The Dartmouth Medical School is still quite orthodox. The nation's fourth oldest, it has had a 2-year program for most of the century until the full 4-year program was reintroduced in the 1970s. Relative to other schools in the study, Dartmouth is in the early throes of change, having only recently begun to review its traditional curriculum. It is new enough to the game that no one yet sees where the boat-rocking will lead. Many question altering the tried and true even one bit. Mission is put cautiously, therefore, allowing for a wide range of possible outcomes.

- The primary mission is to create the right environment in which students will learn about medicine. I have always had a "realistic" view of what medical school is and what these 4 years are. It is the transition between what you were and did before and what you will yet do. It is not an end in itself but a process to translate college graduates into physicians. Our optimal mission therefore is to create a learning environment that in this relatively short period of time leads them into what they will next do. Another way of saying what the mission is, which is what I say to students, is that they are here to acquire facts, skills, attitudes, and values. They are here to learn how to think with facts, how to use skills and to know when not to use various of them, and to adopt some very important attitudes and values. I tell students that it is as important in medical school to learn what you do not know as it is to learn what you do know. In these 4 years of science and preparation for doctoring we introduce issues of problem solving in a way that students usually have not encountered before and, in doing this, I think that we have an opportunity to influence a whole set of physician behaviors. My fundamental premise about the new curriculum, therefore, is that it needs to give students more free time and less structured time. With regard to the Robert Wood Johnson Foundation generalists initiative, even if we do achieve the 50% percent goal of generalists, it still leaves the other 50%, say plus or minus 10. I have a strong belief, now being incorporated into the New Directions Committee, in creating the freedom that will allow all students whatever they are preparing for to experience the broader environment at Dartmouth College. Whether it is a concern for the science of practice or the ethics of the doctor–patient relationship or an interest in the spirit of science, I would like to activate in all our students not only the skills but also the attitudes and values that would make them good doctors.

- The school views itself as committed . . . to giving students the skills and attitudes of a strong generalist, although it is not necessarily focused on producing generalist physicians. [I: Had we been speaking 10 years ago?] My words might have been the same, namely, to provide students a broad general medical education and to prepare them to do residencies, but my conceptual focus has sharpened considerably over the last 4 to 5 years. . . . First, working with students, I think more about mission. Second, the environment is changing. Society needs more generalist physicians. Thus we are trying to find a middle ground between social need and academic content. What has changed is that earlier I would have described the role of the school only in terms of serving the students' needs. Now I describe it in terms of a role of the school in serving both students and societal interests.

- [Mission] is being redefined. . . . Presently we are about to launch an MD–PhD program for a small number of people to become clinical scientists. Of the remainder we want half generalists and half specialists. Neither the dean nor the faculty want to be viewed as a generalist school, though. Schools called generalist are less prestigious. . . . This is not true, of course, inasmuch as the January issue of *Academic Medicine* included the University of California San Francisco among generalist schools! Nevertheless, Dartmouth does not want to be classified along with [generalist schools only]. [I: Has the school's mission changed at all in the last decade?] I have kept track of how many of our students enter specialties and how many primary care, and I can say that there was no attempt prior to the last year's explicit mission-making deal in strategic planning to think about the generalist–specialist mix here. Before this very recent effort, we just asked, "What is the best place with the best track record to send our graduates?" Recently, I wrote both Dean Wallace and Dean Culp and the chairs of medicine and community and family medicine and said, "Great, now that we are committed to 50% generalists, we must rethink the goal of placing our students in high-tech tertiary-care medical centers. These are incompatible with training for generalist care. Our students will have no role models if they go to the Brigham or to Yale and so forth. We must be willing to give up that track record mentality. We must look at programs including those at the University of Washington and University of California San Francisco in primary care medicine and pediatrics or at Mass General in inner-city primary care."

The Harvard Medical School is consistently heterodox. No one way may overarch at Harvard. Each may only be excellent. If innovation at Harvard can never be wholesale, therefore, it may yet be centrally sponsored and as bold as the New Pathway has been since 1985. Like New Mexico, Harvard launched an experimental track, then watched and adjusted it, and, as New Mexico may, Harvard then integrated positive parts of the experiment across the curriculum.[1] Though proportionately fewer faculty at a larger school are affected, contrasting cries arose at Harvard, too, of "watered down!" and "not in my curriculum!" Nowhere has decanal leadership been more important to curricular innovation than at Harvard. The school did not need an educational experiment, after all, to distinguish it from the pack. Mission at Harvard is put in terms as heterodox as the school itself.

- Our mission is to prepare for the medicine of tomorrow through the discovery of new ideas. Even more important is to prepare young people to enter all fields of medicine and medical science. In that spectrum, we do not have a particular focus. Many faculty have argued that we should be research oriented, and of course we are. But the faculty as a whole has rejected such a statement as a single overarching focus. Now we are faced with a strong demand by the federal government that we produce more primary care physicians, that we raise the level of such training. Although we have long had a productive division of primary care, and last year established a new department of ambulatory care and prevention, we have never announced an institutional commitment to provide a certain percentage of each class as primary-care physicians. We aim instead at

---

[1] "The Holmes Society was created at HMS in 1985 by Dean Daniel Tosteson as the home of the 'New Pathway.' Its founding precepts were integrated into the HMS curriculum when we were joined by the three other Societies in 1987 (Castle, Cannon, Peabody) that now have a 'Common Pathway.' The Academic Societies serve as the organizational framework for your medical education, provide a context for social functions that bring faculty and students together, and promote vertical integration of the four years of the curriculum. The Societies consist of students, faculty, and administrative staff. Members of a Society share a Society cluster area and classrooms in the Medical Education Center. Approximately forty students from each class are assigned by lot on admission and remain in the Society during medical/dental school." (From the Oliver Wendell Holmes Society *Program Guide*, Harvard Medical School, 1991–1992.)

educating individual leaders in whatever kind of medicine
or medical science they choose to practice. The issue is
whether we can actually achieve this, whether we can develop the four societies into four departments of general
medical education. In every dimension that you can imagine, in the *n*-dimensional space of contemporary medicine,
change is occurring at an accelerating rate. The most important of these changes has to do with the disciplines in
the natural sciences that bear on medicine. These will
shape the fundamental ways that we look at and think
about ourselves as human beings. But I also do not want to
underestimate the power of the economy and society and
the need to reorganize medical services. A crisis in the way
medical services are organized is upon us, and it is visibly
distorting the environment in which medical education
and research takes place. These changes raise the question
of how we will finance the rising cost of medicine in the future. [I: Have you changed your view of the school's mission
during your tenure here?] Not much, but I have learned a
lot! You have probably asked a lot of people about the New
Pathway. For me it is not problem based per se, nor, for that
matter, any particular new idea. Indeed, almost everything
that we are exploring here has been done at other times in
the past or is now being done somewhere else as well. Almost all the verbiage and ideas that we have tried to express concretely you can find already in the 1920s. For me,
the New Pathway is the commitment of our faculty to
search continuingly for new and better ways to educate
medical students in a rapidly changing environment.

The University of California, San Francisco, School of Medicine (UCSF) is bimodal. Like private Harvard, public UCSF
ranks among top research schools and recruits the very best biomedical and clinical faculty and students. A bargain for the latter compared to the privates, UCSF outdraws all but Harvard.
Unlike Harvard, it graduates half its MD classes in primary
care, a result not of any new pathway but of schoolwide admissions policy and curriculum development efforts. Demography,
in a state whose population exceeds 20 million and is the most
varied in the nation, favors student body diversity. Bimodality,

in high-tech/low-tech, specialist/generalist, research/clinical medicine, one or the other side of which pleases some and perplexes others, is a recurrent theme in mission statements.

- [Our mission] is bimodal. It is to be at the cutting edge of the biomedical sciences and to train clinical practitioners for the state. Turning out subspecialists is not our mission, although we have produced our share. When [our new dean], who was conceived as being primarily interested in biomedical science, came in, there was a real fear that he would change admissions policy to that end. He appointed [a] former chair of the department of medicine as chair of admissions and we were initially afraid that the school would begin to look only at 4.0s in the sciences, that all our students would have to be MD–PhD candidates or the equivalent. But this did not happen. The admissions committee strengthened the student body but did not change its composition otherwise. We continued to attract a very diverse student body, representing this very big diverse state. We have also promoted primary care, but without that being widely recognized in view of UCSF's scientific strength. Our student body comes from all over the world. Seventy percent are on financial aid, even with our low tuition.
- The mission is to turn out first-rate physicians, not just for California but for the entire United States, to do front-line research, and—but only incidentally—to provide services and patient care. We do 40% of the inpatient care in San Francisco and 40% of the emergency care in the city. Thus we are rather balanced in our output. We have a high proportion of primary-care physicians. About 50% of our graduates go into primary care. The big question, of course, is downstream: How many stay in primary care?
- The basic mission is to train physicians for society in the broadest sense, but this may not always be in the forefront of our attention. [I: Who is overlooking it?] The faculty as a whole, because of the enormous impact of research and research accomplishments. This focus has tended to take center stage with education as a lesser priority. As a member of the National Academy of Sciences, everyone thought

that I would be dominated by a focus on research. But it became clear to me very soon that education needed a much stronger emphasis here.

The two Canadian schools are new and smaller public institutions, like New Mexico and Hawaii. They also resemble their U.S. counterparts in how fundamentally innovative they are. They differ markedly between themselves, however, in where they stand in the change process. Thus McMaster very early, at its founding in the 1960s in fact, and Sherbrooke very late, fighting for its life and by sweeping conversion in the mid-1980s, created fully problem-based curricula with strong community and population orientation.

The McMaster University Faculty of Health Sciences MD program is at a crossroads. Founded under Toronto's shadow in the 1960s, at the very start of the current reform cycle, McMaster became and remained a recognized leader in problem-based community-oriented learning, sending envoys out into the world to share the new way. By now, an old guard that wants to preserve that way confronts a new guard that wants to follow new rules. A few reject the polarity and want to apply the old method to adapt to the school's new situation. Describing MD program mission, therefore, some reaffirm the legacy in methods and perspectives for which McMaster became well known in the 1970s, whereas others think that what actually drives faculty and program is the research- and clinic-revenue imperative that came in during the 1980s.

- [Our mission] is to provide degree programs for students in the health professions and undertake health research. Fifteen years ago, . . . I would have said that our mission was interprofessional, community oriented, innovative, and based on a progressive function that was much more apparent than it is today. Fifteen years ago, there was a much more dynamic sense, and we were smaller. [I: Why has the program changed?] First of all, size. Second, the people here are now much older. Third, there has been a major shift in funding of clinical faculty as a result of declining fiscal support from government for education. Thus in 1986, a new practice plan was instituted that put more value on clinical services at the cost of education programs. The school's values, therefore, have become more focused on clinical earnings. The critical moment was 1986, because the practice plan committee in effect changed the value system of clinical faculty here.

- It is to produce practitioners ready to go into residency training with primarily a health care delivery orientation and the capacity to enter any field of medicine. The mission is also that they will take with them certain attitudes . . . that are more holistic in their approach to patient care. Here we very much emphasize communication and the family and community context of patients. In 1982, the description of the mission that I just gave was first published and became policy. It reflected the policies of the late 1960s and the founding of the MD program here. [I: Has there been any change over the decade?] There is an increased focus through unit 5 on the community and on population. This has come since 1984. [I: And what was the impetus for that?] Well, we actually blocked out a unit in 1982. It was poorly defined and called the "Life Cycle Unit." As it evolved, it took a community focus. It is a 12–week block between clerkships, which deals with life-cycle issues. Students go out into a community, conduct interviews, map the community, and so forth. They begin visiting patients, for example, in chronic care settings or industry centers. And there is an expectation that they will follow up. . . . But 10 years ago, the MD program was also more central to the faculty's thoughts. . . . My fear now is that it is peripheral to what people really want to do here. It was harder and harder the last 2 years, for example, to find tutors for the program.

- To promote education and research through student-based, self-directed learning, with reference to the health of society. [I: Had we been speaking 8 to 10 years ago?] One difference would have been my focus on the word "health" and its meaning. In the last 3 to 4 years here the notion of health and of all its determinants has become much more preeminent than before. Thus while my wording might have included health care before, it would have been health care centered on the traditional role of the health care professional. Now I would say that health is a broader concept that takes into account other relevant systems, including social support systems, employment, as well as social marketing relative to health. In this sense, health care professionals do not have all the expertise, and now we are aware of this. This broader sense of health and health care may also be translated, I see now, into the notion of a social contract. The only debate centers around the time frame for that contract and who determines the contract. Universities have traditionally assumed that they have the right to define the contract, but now society is wanting to define these terms. This is shocking to the university and to medical education professionals, but I believe that the truth is somewhere in the middle.

The University of Sherbrooke Faculty of Medicine is only just embarking on reform. With talk of a closing in the recessionary early 1980s, Quebec's youngest and smallest medical faculty changed across-the-board from a very traditional curriculum to an entirely problem-based curriculum. The dean saw that the faculty had quickly to distinguish itself from three, more established, provincial medical faculties or face closure, and so recruited a problem-based learning messiah to engineer a change-over that worked, in part because no one doubted either man's resolve. But if Sherbrooke utterly redefined teaching method in the mid-1980s, it also maintained its mission largely unaltered.

- [Our mission is] to prepare doctors in connection with the real needs of the population. This was one of the main reasons for the reform. Even if the faculty says that the mission here is research, our main reason for being is to treat the people for the problems that they have. We are not here primarily to treat people for what we want them to have. [I: Had we been speaking 8 to 10 years ago?] No difference. This is one subject about which I did not change my mind. We are a small university; we have to compete against big universities. We need people with a real sense of the importance of what we do, people with a strong commitment and a feeling of ownership of the medical faculty here. Our school was built here in the 1960s out of nothing. It came out of politics and out of vision. It was founded largely by people dissatisfied with the research and typical service orientation of the University of Montreal. Many of the people first involved with Sherbrooke were French Canadians who had studied at the Mayo Clinic in Rochester. We have always had a strong sense of ownership and commitment at this school. When the school was founded, many of the French Canadians at the Mayo Clinic came back. The primary dissatisfaction concerned what a teaching hospital and a university hospital should be. Now they are integrated everywhere, but in 1968–1970 they were very separated. Now our model has become quite widespread, for example, at the Universities of Edmonton and Calgary where the scientific, clinical, educational, and other health professional programs are put all together. So, our mission really is the same as it was at the beginning. If anything, we now give more response to the community and to social problems. This was there right at the founding, however.

- [Mission is] to cover three classical areas. First, education, to train physicians needed by Quebec, to center their education on social needs; second, research; and third, of course, services. Now, about the educational mission, it is first and foremost social. We train 25 subspecialty programs for the community. Beyond the MD, we offer the MS and the PhD in seven disciplines. We also offer courses of study in nursing and in the basic sciences at the baccalaureate level. This campus was in fact created to produce physicians for Quebec. . . . If you look at the proportion of general care such as family medicine and pediatrics and specialized care or research physicians that we turn out, 55% of our graduates are in the former area and 45% percent in the latter. They are spread out over the entire province of Quebec, not just in the university cities. Physician distribution is not a problem therefore. We are cited as the school that produces for the whole province. [I: Had we been speaking 8 to 10 years ago?] It has remained fairly constant. Recently, in fact, we pulled out the mission statement that was written in 1969 and we discovered happily that it was almost identical to the one that we had rewritten in the last several years.

- [Mission is] to educate nondifferentiated physicians who can be accepted into subspecialty or family practice or research careers in medicine. Those were the goals 10 years ago, too. But their implementation differs now. And access to specialties was easier then than now. . . . We are a public institution and access to residency is under government rules. The provincial government has decided these matters for at least 10 years. The mix is 50% in specialty medicine and 50% in family medicine. This is policy. It is very interesting that in 1969 when the faculty of medicine was just getting under way we had a framework for goals at Sherbrooke. Then, last year, we had a presentation with the administration. I went back to get the framework statement, and I discovered that roughly the same goals as now were in the 1969 statement. The only way that they differed at all was that in 1969 Sherbrooke wanted an earlier differentiation of medical students in the program, for example, by giving some academic experience in the first year. The other goals were exactly the same, for example, those concerning humanistic qualities and community orientation of our graduates.

- It is what we call formative education, more than the transmission of knowledge. The mission is likewise to serve the community, . . . the province of Quebec as well. For me, the school is not devoted enough to the community, even now. [I: Had we been speaking 8 or 10 years ago?] There has really been a move over this period. Around 1985–1986, we moved rapidly after we became conscious that we had to be more community oriented. Before, our mission was "science." It was that our students should be optimally knowledgeable. It was very important for us to produce the "best students" in terms of knowledge. For a good part of the faculty now, the emphasis is on medical humanism. Two-thirds of them will mention this now, even though only one-half will actually act on it. [In contrast] we are not really very far along with respect to the community orientation yet. One of the problems is that, although the undergraduate program may have changed . . . it is still not the whole faculty. The graduate faculty is much less aware of our new orientation. They are not against it, but there is little reflection on the meaning of this at the graduate level. It is only just starting. Our emphasis on humanistic medical education and on community development will have a lot of implications at the graduate level, for example, in research. Their orientation now is what ours was before 1985–1986, namely, to produce the "best researchers" . . . the same orientation as a big faculty of medicine in the United States toward research, and this does have an effect on undergraduate training here at Sherbrooke.

CHAPTER 2

Major Problems

The problem at new, little-endowed Mercer is financial stability. Indeed the school would be doubting its viability even after more than a decade's operation if it were not for a Georgia-insider dean's bid for "formula" funding from the state and for a better deal from the university. The quid pro quo from the legislature, adamantly adhered to at Mercer, is that graduates remain mission compliant.

- Two problems. The first is financial. We went from $4.5 million to $8 million annually from the state, but then the state, because of financial difficulties, cut us back $700,000 over the last 2 years. The governor has now recommended restoring that [sum] in the next year's budget. The drop strongly concerned our accreditors. My concern now is that we do not yet have a "funding formula" from the state. The second problem concerns the school's mission. It has to be always out there. This is a human business and not 100% of our graduates will choose residencies in our six primary care disciplines. And not 100% of those residents will practice in the state and in areas of need. Therefore the question becomes, how much attention to put on mission? We have had to date about 4% a year of our graduates choose nonmission-compliant residencies. That may not sound like much, but I ask myself, What if that number doubles? [I: Had we been speaking 6 or 7 years ago?] Then the problem was to prove to the [accreditation] committee that we are capable of educating medical students. There was doubt at the time. In the 1980s I was pushed, first of all, to prove that we could educate medical students and, second of all, to stay mission constant. Now, in the 1990s, having established these two things, we can begin to branch out. Keeping to our mission, we have been helped by two things that were not at all in our control. First of all, the need for primary-care physicians has become a national matter. Both the AAMC [American Association of Medical Colleges] and the AMA [American Medical Association] are worried and talking about this. We were ahead of the group, as it turned out, fortunately. Second, there has been a wave of dissent with the way curriculum is delivered in medical schools. This launched the whole interest in problem-based learning.

When I came to Mercer, they said to me at Emory, "The only way that you will make Mercer work is to abolish the problem-based curriculum." First, I do not believe that I could have done so. Second, I do not believe that I should have. [I: What would you propose for the future with respect to the second 2 years of the Mercer undergraduate medical education program?] I do not see major problems with the second 2 years. I have always felt that bedside teaching is very similar to the first 2 years of the problem-based learning concept. There is a natural linkage between the two. We do need more systematic analysis of problem-based learning in the second 2 years, however. A larger question, in my view, is how we use elective time. I believe that our mission is very tied to what is referred to as population-based medicine and that we ought to use the curriculum for more issues in population-based medicine. Thus I believe that we ought to examine our current elective offerings with this in mind and link these offerings to mission. The students who drift from the school's mission have often used the electives to shop for a super-specialty. The curriculum committee and the academic dean are currently reviewing the electives program for attachment to mission.

• Right now ... the biggest problem is money. This has partly to do with the national economy and partly with Mercer's difficulty. The law school and medical school at Mercer have been heavily taxed to support the undergraduate college program. We are the rich kids on the block. We got cut last year because of retrenchment in the state budget. Naturally, the university did not help with the shortfall, even though when it is restored the university will take its share! Fifty percent of the new money coming into the university next year will be medical school money. Happily we developed a mission that now seems to be fully compliant with the national movement to primary care. The national student loan policy in this regard, for example, really helps us, whereas it hurts many other medical schools. It is so well timed that Mercer may become a regional primary-care center and receive over a million dollars in Area Health Education Center money. [Ten years ago,] the first problems we faced were accreditation and getting the school started. Money was not a problem. The problem was convincing people to buy into problem-based learning, to attract senior faculty willing to come, to get research started. I do not think that there are many medical schools that graduate their charter class as well as we did. We graduated a high number of our charter class of 24.

At Hawaii, in the midst of a top-down changeover to problem-based learning, the problem is to consolidate a change that has left some basic scientists far behind. As their counterparts at New Mexico fear they will be, in merging the primary care and traditional curricula, so the basic scientists at Hawaii fear they have been curricularly disempowered by problem-based learning. Eliminating basic science courses in favor of an untried pedagogy still shocks some faculty several years after the fact.

- The curriculum [is the problem]. It is something that we need to continue to discuss and to work on and get consensus on. The initial shock is wearing off, but even so there continues to be a lot of change. Even now there is a lot of revolutionary change being proposed and implemented. This ferment will continue. [I: Which divisions among faculty are most prominent in the curriculum debate?] I would say first of all that the impetus for change was with the dean and with two or three other faculty. There was a significant number of faculty who felt and feel that this was not a good thing to do. [I: Was it the speed of change or the change per se?] All of the above. It was the philosophy itself of problem-based learning and the elimination of all the basic science courses! It is an entirely different way of teaching and there is a lot of insecurity. The idea that from day one you can jump in right in the middle with a given problem in pathology or pharmacology was felt to be a little crazy. It really was a different way to learn. Some faculty felt that it was nonsystematic coverage of the material. They felt that students were not being instructed enough in the basic sciences. There was quite a bit of that sort of feeling, a lot of concern about how well the basic sciences were being taught. When it was first introduced, moreover, faculty were told that it would not take more teaching time. For many this turned out to be completely untrue. [Ten years ago,] the perennial problem was available funds from the state and the federal government as well as problems funding research grants. That has not changed! At the time, the curriculum was not anything we were talking about. [I: Has curriculum change worsened research grant-getting capacity?] No, I cannot say that, but we are all much busier than we were before. There was trouble with funding before, and there is still trouble. The change is that the new curriculum does mean that you are diverted to some extent.

I want to reemphasize that I am not all negative about problem-based learning. There are some positive things. In my view, what we should have is a hybrid, for example, in the first year a traditional didactic program and then in the second year problem-based learning. I would be all in favor of that. Students need background in basic science material to go into problem-based learning. They need a foundation on which then they may go into greater detail and depth. The chair of pharmacology at Michigan State complains that he only has 50 lectures! If we had 50 lectures it would be something! My guess is that with the New Pathway, Harvard gives half the number of lectures that it did before. The problem we have at the moment here is that there is a cadre of people who feel that pure problem-based learning is the only way to go. Hopefully, we will be able to fine tune, and we are doing it to some extent now. We do have Wednesday conferences and Friday colloquia, and many of these wind up being lectures. [I: And students want them?] Yes. And there are a couple of hours for lab work on Wednesdays. Still, it is not a system, it is a mish-mash. We need to convince the curriculum people to change this.

Disaffection in anticipation of change—polarization before, not after, the fact—is the problem at New Mexico. The experiment has long been safely tracked at New Mexico in a primary care curriculum parallel to the traditional. Merging the two, New Mexico now meets the sort of dismay among basic scientists seen at Hawaii, even as it recounts a wider range of difficulties—the state's competitive health care environment, difficult relations with the university, overcommitted faculty, departmentalism—more typical of bigger schools like Minnesota.

• Like every every medical school today, we face real competition for faculty resources spread among patient care, research, and education obligations, though it is less of a problem here as all of us are on a strict full-time regimen. The state gives us a contract for fixed salaries no matter what else we earn. . . . But right now the major issue is curriculum revision. There is opposition, and some faculty do not see ownership of the new curriculum, see it being shoved through by the so-called radicals in the primary-care unit. For example, a chair in the division of surgery told us that some faculty might decide not to award the MD to students in the primary-care program. It is getting back at us for having a primary-care orientation. Then too, there is rapid change going on in the medical-care delivery system in the state. Who knows what impact that will have on us. We are a small hospital dependent on all kinds of support. (On November 3, the county will pass or not pass a levy that will directly affect our ability to operate. On our behalf we have argued that we see a much broader spectrum of patients from every social or economic group, that our students get a better view than the private hospitals can offer, and that we have a better mix of patients and educational experiences.) Then there is the question of leadership of the academic health center here. It is an ongoing battle between the hospital and the dean of the medical school, who is also director of the medical center. It is the typical conflict. The president wants to take a look at reorganizing the medical school. The president wants to divest the university of the hospital and wants a vice president for health affairs separate from the office of the dean. But the fact is there ain't many health affairs here, other than the university hospital. There is only a small nursing school, pharmacy school, and a school of dental hygiene.

• [Increasingly] there is the issue of looking at medical education in 4–year compared to 7– to 9– to 10–year terms, of educating medical students at the same time that you educate hospital house staff. Right now the two parts are too segmented and the accrediting agencies of graduate medical education are looking more closely at this segmentation. There needs to be more effective communication among faculties . . . about opening the gates between levels. For too long now at this school, although we did not start off this way, we have become more and more departmentalized, adding and subtracting the various departments' hours in the curriculum. When the school started off in 1964, it was organ oriented and biology based. About 1972, it became more departmentally organized so that anatomy had this time slot and biochemistry had that time slot. When I participate in accreditation site visits, I have noticed the way chairs define their first needs, for example, in clinical departments in terms of fellows, house staff, and only then, medical students. Basic science chairs, in turn, define their needs in terms of postdocs, graduate students, and only then in terms of medical students. Here the primary care curriculum has given a big impetus to faculty to examine medical education first of all from an intellectual point of view. I have tried to say to faculty and to the departments that medical students are the base of medical education. I have tried to tell them that the state government in Santa Fe wants to know what we are doing for medical students first of all. Thus the traditional faculty, who look at the curriculum in terms of my nine lectures and yours, have had to ask, "What are we actually trying to do?" My role in this has been to be a skeptic, to remind people that neither the primary-care curriculum nor the traditional curriculum is immortal, to question both approaches, to suggest that maybe you do not need a lecture here or a tutorial there, to say that both groups can learn from the other. This all goes back to the idea of not repressing the gene for humility.

At big, public, department-driven Minnesota, the problem is not too much but too little schoolwide education policy, not too many but too few efforts at curriculum integration and coordination, not too much but too little central leadership. At the same time, the school experiences too little autonomy from universitywide educational policy in matters of promotion and tenure.

- [The] number one [problem] is to get the clinical department heads, of whom there are 17 or 18, to share power in terms of the greater good of the institution, to recognize that the whole is greater than the sum of the parts. It will not happen if they stick to their little islands, to their shared practice plans. They need to establish common educational goals. By the way, this is the contrast between this place and the Mayo Medical School. Here it is much more entrepreneurial and department oriented. At Mayo, there is a tradition of sacrificing to the greater good. [Here] if there were more sharing, it would lead to more of a sense of corporate responsibility for the medical education of students . . . more role modeling and excellence in teaching students. Now it is individual glory. It is, "I am the premier person in field X or Y." We must shift from individual glory to explicit excellence in the institution. Mayo did this by focusing on the corporate good, pooling resources, and getting the best educators they could. They also have been good at giving time off from clinics for research or educational enterprise. Our last dean said that the strength of this institution compared to the Mayo was that we had an every-person-for-himself attitude here. What is plainly true, however, is that the top-down approach, the direction-from-above approach, is not adapted at all to Minnesota. [I: Had we spoken 8 to 10 years ago?] It would have been largely the same problem then, although it has become worse since 1982. Interestingly, what has made the same problem worse since then is that the context has changed. Nowadays the way business is being done with medicine in society, it is much more organized and contractual. Thus the problem, namely, our very individualist ethic, is much more obvious.

- In my view, it is lack of interest in medical education and lack of leadership in the principled oversight of the curriculum. In the latter, we have benign neglect for the most part. [I: What proportion benign neglect, what proportion lack of principled oversight?] It is 90% neglect. [I: Where does that leave you?] Needing to satisfy myself with small, incremental victories or satisfactions.

- Our relationship to the rest of the university [is a problem]. Medical schools always have particular problems in financial, personnel, and faculty management areas. We need more flexibility in responding to our financial restrictions and in dealing directly with the start-up of our cancer center and our primary-care initiative, for example. In both of these matters, we have to go through the university president's office, and it would be far better if we could manage them ourselves. I would also say that there are issues in personnel management, for example, in the probationary period required before tenure. The period of time given in the rest of the university is insufficient to allow faculty in medicine to gain sufficient experience and records of productivity. The AAUP [American Association of University Professors] system, after all, of 6 + 1 years was established in 1913!

The problem at previous-cycle innovator Case Western Reserve, as at McMaster, is the tension between past and present. As with mission, so the school's major problem is defined in strongly contrasting terms, respectively, that too few and too many resources are being expended on general professional education relative to other activities. If Minnesota were a smaller, less far-flung school, it might presently feature as pronounced a conflict as Case Western Reserve's between past education legacy and current research- and clinic-revenue imperative.

- Ultimately [the problem] is financial. If you have the money, you can do a lot. All sorts of subsets of that statement are true, too. I have a personal view probably not shared by most faculty that if we want to educate "blast" physicians, we can do this much more inexpensively than it is now being done. In fact the major educational expense here is to provide a kind of menu of opportunities in which few students actually participate. This is paralleled at the university level by the expense entailed in offering 10 to 20 different language programs. This school has a tremendous number of full-time faculty, up to 1,100, in fact. We are highest in faculty–student ratio in the United States, and although we do not pay a lot in faculty salaries directly, there are a lot of perks. A different structure would be far less expensive if you wanted just to train "blast" physicians. I have the notion that in a school like this where the average age of students is 26, it might be easier than elsewhere for students to have an idea of their career plans upon entry. [I: And with more clarity by students earlier, there would not be as much need for a menu approach to the curriculum?] Yes, and you would be further along in your training by the time you finished medical school, or further along with graduate studies. Because I was an oriental affairs major in college, I have the notion that medical students do not enter medical studies without already having some knowledge of history, philosophy, ethics, and so forth. Thus it is not really so that they have to start all over again with a broad extramedical formation here. Medical school after all is not a great place to teach ethics.
- The major problems [in the 1950s] were, first, how do you expand and legitimize the roles of the basic science departments? Second, how do you encourage and recognize basic research in the clinical departments? Third, how do you generate people adept at basic science and clinical medicine, as opposed to one or the other? In those days the idea that one could be a splendid investigator, clinician, and teacher was the accepted doctrine. This is no longer true. Now if you have an NIH [National Institutes of Health] grant, your academic life depends on renewing it—your salary, your appointment, your tenure, your promotion, all depend on re-

newing grants. If you are a clinician, all this depends on your practice income. This is the case at Lakeside Hospital already, and it is closing in on faculty at the Metropolitan, Veterans Administration, and Mt. Sinai Hospitals. One of the things that I hesitate to bring up with our chair in the department of medicine . . . exactly concerns this problem. I believe that he neglects the fact that the guy who gets a 3– to 4–year NIH grant and then a renewal for 5 more years will very likely run out of gas in 12 years or so. Sooner or later, his ability to be in the forefront will go away. The problem is that you cannot just discard these people who are, in any case, more transient than you think in the long run. But I do not know how it should be done otherwise. I do not know how to achieve persistent excellence. I do know, however, that to encourage excellence in the medical community requires openness and time for discussion and that this is becoming more and more rare.

Dartmouth's problem is deep ambivalence about change, the cross-product of demoralization, self-doubt, a sense of unrealized potential, and compensatory idealization of a simpler past. Dartmouth is a smaller 4–year school in a big league, insufficiently endowed to keep the Ivies company as it once did as their 2–year feeder school.

- Money is the problem. A significant portion of our funding comes from tuition, approximately 10%. Another 25 to 30% comes from indirect research support. Patient care comes in at about 20% and money from endowment, gifts, grants, and contracts brings in the remainder, up to 50%. This all totals $134 million a year. Even so we are looking at a $3–10 million deficit next year unless we increase the contribution from patient care. At a place this size, I have tried to convince our dean that research never pays for itself. To get a high-powered chairman of chemistry, we recently had to offer a multimillion dollar package. With a 55% indirect cost recovery from the federal government, you never really recoup these outlays. The only way to recoup or to break even is if you are lucky enough to have prodigies among faculty who become principal investigators on research sponsored by the National Institutes of Health and bring in a lot of indirect research money. This way you would not have to bring big shots already with big reputations.

- This is a school that has had for some period of time a lot of potential that has not been realized. The reason [for this] is related partly to past experiences in which the school developed something very strong only to lose it. From a historical point of view, the school has a scar that really frames the psychology of the place. You could call it the molecular biology crisis of the 1960s. That was a time when the medical school was a very distinguished center for molecular biology research. That program was very much in keeping with the tradition at Dartmouth of being a basic-science teaching institution. We were a 2–year medical school, after all, until very recently. In the late 1960s, for reasons of personality and vision, there was a collision between the basic science dimension and the emerging clinical emphasis here. And the basic-science people lost, in effect, and a number of nationally recognized people went elsewhere. They left behind them a sense that the institution had to choose between basic-science and clinical programs. This is a profoundly wrong perception of how the Dartmouth Medical School will move forward, but it became the sense of the place. At the same time, faculty came to think that it was difficult or impossible to do something distinguished here. They adopted the view that we were once great but that we cannot maintain it here. Related to this is the problem, which follows from being a small school, that, if you do have a distinguished program, it will almost always be based on one or two people. These few people in turn often have many options, and the problem is that you tend to lose them. In a way I am amazed that we keep so many. But when we do lose one, it is always interpreted within this historical context and understanding that we cannot maintain the distinction that we once had. Thus our major current problem at the Dartmouth Medical School is self-confidence. We need to develop a better sense of confidence in our ability to do something distinguished. This plays out as concern over a number of things. First, resources. Second, governance. Third, simultaneously accomplishing a number of dimensions.

- If someone gave me $6 million, we could have an education program here that would knock your socks off. Even $2 million if it were for education, real teaching and learning, would be a godsend. [I: Would you have defined the major problem of the school similarly had I asked the same question 10 years ago?] Yes, but I would not have known what I know now. I would have said that you are punished if you teach, but I would not have known quite why. Teaching here, like elsewhere, is done on your own time, is unpaid. This has not changed.

The problem at Harvard has been to maintain momentum for New Pathway innovation—primary and ambulatory care instruction, doctor–patient communication, health promotion and disease prevention, clinical and basic science integration, problem-based learning, population perspective—within an institution otherwise dominated by advanced biomedical research and at a time of schoolwide funding cuts.

- At this school ... there have been across-the-board cutbacks at every level [so that] everybody has suffered somewhat. Even though the school is private and has a large endowment and a large research base ... the fact is still negative. It will not help, and it will hurt. The trend will especially interfere with those physicians who have clinical teaching responsibilities in the wards and also work in outpatient settings. Across-the-board cuts mean that practitioners who are already struggling to make a living will be harder to find and to train to teach.
- [By the mid-1980s, some of us wanted] to move students into ambulatory settings and to teach these subjects. It was part of [our] view that an ambulatory care clerkship should be established. [Dean] Federman led it as a new required clerkship to last 8 weeks to put students in ambulatory settings. There was some resistance from the faculty, but it was then reluctantly accepted by the faculty. By the time the New Pathway was implemented, it was a requirement. A Kaiser grant supported our effort to move into primary-

care settings. Then there was the 3-year patient–doctor course, originally set up for the New Pathway. Its major goal was, beginning with week one, to have students meet patients. Both the Kaiser grant and the patient–doctor course immediately operated to shift students into primary-care settings. Then too [Dean] Tosteson wanted change. He promised reform. It was in the air. So it was not only the Kaiser grant. [Still] I would like to see expansion of the patient–doctor course content, for example, to every other week with ambulatory patients. I want to enhance this contact, to a panel of patients or to a family right from the start—say, if a student were to follow a pregnant mom for 4 years or an elderly couple or a group of teenagers or a terminally ill person—as they do at Case Western Reserve. Now it is just a taste, window shopping. Our leaders have to get closer to their customers. It is a real plus that Harvard has established a preventive ambulatory care practice department [but we still] have to keep working to get to our customers, to where medical practice is really going. . . . For example, in putting a recent grant together to create new generalists, it did not occur to our academic leaders to invite HMO [health maintenance organization] leaders in the Boston area into the conversation. They need to be brought into a conversation. Therefore we need more of a community of academic leaders . . . of curriculum directors, deans, hospital heads. But we also need heads of ambulatory care centers, neighborhood health clinics, and HMOs. They are not visible enough yet.

• My perception is that in the first 2 years of teaching, basic science faculty would like nothing better than to have issues like disease prevention and health promotion pushed off into a separate parallel occasional course because, they think, these have nothing to do with biochemistry and molecular biology. The message given to students is that it is secondary, does not matter, except to the converted. But, if you could imagine ways to integrate these issues of prevention and so forth into the discipline and learning of biomedical science, then they would take on firmer weight and vitality. The fact is that if teachers are not going to integrate them, then the students definitely will not. There are a few sporadic cases involving individual personalities. The process of breaking each entering class into small groups for tutorials has allowed some individual expressions of interests in these areas. Instead of a one-person lecture format taught by someone who does not care, the tutorials have given students some exposure to teachers who do care about integrating material. But there are no collective efforts [in this direction].

A big proportion of students expresses interest in primary care at the beginning, but then few actually enter it. If one could fertilize that interest in the beginning and integrate it with the rest of science, it would help a lot. The prevailing attitude at Harvard is that this is a soft, undesirable part of medicine, primary care that is, that it is not really the mission of the school. A really hard-core reductionist researcher believes that all we have to do is wait for the kids to grow up and they will see the light. Then, we will leave primary care for other schools. [But this is] bad for Harvard and for what I see to be the most pressing needs of our society. I do not see a pressing need at the moment to prolong life. I do see the need for resources and strong emphasis on delivering health care to the underserved.

• Problem-based learning uses clinical experience as a vehicle for stimulating learning, for getting students struggling with real human dilemmas. You could imagine basic science, after all, that has no relationship to clinical medicine, for example, as relates to industrial problems. Here problem-based learning is associated with the patient–doctor course and with early clinical experience, both of which also combine basic and clinical science. Vertical integration stimulates learning in both blocks . . . highlights the complex richness of medicine and exposes students to careers . . . empowers students who now learn more personal skills . . . facilitates early identification of problems, personal and programmatic. [I: Has there been anything wrong with problem-based learning at Harvard?] When faculty are not well trained, it can be a disaster. It can be destructive to students, which equals poor learning. In exit interviews at the end of 2 years, we learned that students in the badly managed groups felt put down, confused, and undermined by the interpersonal components of those groups. Some anxiety is healthy, but it can get to be too much.

- People say you cannot teach empathy . . . but I disagree. It can be done badly, sloppily, or with a lot of heart. People are working very hard here trying to refine the teaching of communication skills with patients. But how do you measure [these] skills anyway? And what are these personal qualities? Curriculum at Harvard changes year by year. I think that it has now become more rigid and that time slots have gotten too filled up. But there is still a current here to keep things going, under the new organization in societies. I see the societies as a place where the curriculum will constantly change. People work extremely hard at innovative teaching here.

- In its first years the New Pathway was very intensive, and students' introduction to clinical medicine, to interviewing or to the physical exam, for example, was spread out over the first 2 years. Then it was changed and, in fact, compromised, and these subjects were spread only over the second year and especially in the last 3 months. One problem with the patient-doctor course at first was that it set up a curriculum that could not be staffed. It took too many bodies to do it. But the biggest problem was that the course caused a row when, to implement it, they had to take apart the established introduction to clinical medicine [ICM] courses. By the mid-1980s many people had spent much effort upgrading these courses and had been very successful. Many thought that the ICM courses were being taken apart on ideological grounds only because of the new idea that clinical training ought to go on longitudinally. People said, "Look, the ICM works, why change it?" The ICM directors were heads of medicine in a number of the big hospitals like Mass General. This was one of the things that led to big resistance to the New Pathway reform. There was considerable resistance to the reform centered in both the clinics and the basic-science departments. Remember that the New Pathway at Harvard was not a late-1960s but a mid-1980s reform and that this recent round of curriculum reform, profound in certain ways, came in only because of how undeniably bad medical education has come to appear. It was all based on a critique of standard medical education that came from the American Association of Medical Colleges' laying claim in the 1980s for why things should be changed by criticizing everything that came before. Here at Harvard then, everyone who had devoted time to teaching, for example, in the ICM course, felt that the reasons given for curriculum reform were a direct criticism of them personally. Thus the dean never managed to capture the idealism of more than a small number of people. No more than 20 or 30 faculty became deeply involved and invested in curriculum reform, although many were politic enough to support it. Only a few people were open and explicit in their criticism throughout. Around the hospitals, there has been widespread quiet resistance.

The problem at UCSF, where so much else is in place, is space, physical and psychological, and it has been for some time. The school makes the hill upon which it is perched look top-heavy. The sense of confinement is palpable. An old agreement to stick to a defined number of square feet severely limits present options, as does a recent city ordinance forbidding labs above the third floor. UCSF is an ant farm running out of alcoves for teaching, research, and patient care alike, just as it has become distinguished in all these pursuits.

• [Our major problem is,] in a word, space, and not just for medical education. The problem of physical space dominates all planning here. About 15 years ago when we built the new hospital and dental school buildings, there was considerable conflict with the neighborhood concerning our growth. As a result the chancellor agreed that we would not expand beyond 3.5 million square feet on this site. It seemed a safe space ceiling then, but now we have bumped up against it. Thus we are increasingly forced to disperse our academic activities around town. We now have large research activities at San Francisco General Hospital, the V.A. Medical Center, and more are planned at Mount Zion. [I: Had we been speaking 8 to 10 years earlier?] I would have said that academic space was our major problem then too, and second, speaking as the chair of the department of medicine, maintaining cohesion and a common sense of purpose in a huge department and extended house staff.

- There are severe crises here of space and of money. This school is inner-city. It grew up from the University of California, but has had difficulty in gaining a separate identity from Berkeley. A few basic scientists, pathologists especially, began to arrive in the 1940s, and others followed in the 1950s. With new leadership in the 1960s the school began to grow rapidly in both size and quality and began for the first time to have national aspirations. With the arrival of Bill Ritter from the University of Washington, the basic sciences began to be renovated. By the late 1970s and early 1980s, UCSF emerged in the top three or four medical schools nationally, depending on whom you asked. In the late 1970s the school had to submit to a numeric square foot limit of 3.315 million square feet of building space on this site because of neighborhood opposition to our recent expansion. That limit seemed sufficient at the time, but the limit was hit already by 1984. Ever since, we have been severely handicapped in space. Faculty are scattered widely in San Francisco with buses scuttling about everywhere. The problem is that you have got to build up here on Parnassus or move out. [I: And the problem 8 to 10 years ago?] Our chancellor bought the Laurel Heights facility, a former insurance building, in order to alleviate our space problems. It seemed a good move at the time, but enormous opposition developed from the neighborhood and we have been in court concerning it ever since. Therefore the space problem has continued to linger.
- First, clinical instruction is so spread out. Most teaching is done by house staff, and you cannot initiate new kinds of teaching in that environment. Eventually, however, some of the house staff and junior faculty will be people trained in problem-based learning and ambulatory care settings. They themselves will demand change in how to teach medical students in clerkships. Other problems, perhaps the biggest, are cost and efficiency. You can only learn so much from standardized patients. So less is happening here, in clinical instruction, because of our highly decentralized ur-

ban location and related difficulty in terms of the quality of teaching in clinical settings. Frankly I am pessimistic about seminal changes occuring in clinical teaching in our current inpatient services.

The Canadians' problems contrast as age does to youth. McMaster's is the problem of accretion, a long-standing innovator's not knowing quite how to reinvent itself, having so often and so well served to reinvent others. MD program troubles—biomedical science content in tutorial, nonexpert versus expert tutors, isolation in a health sciences faculty, preserving the population perspective, growing numbers of strictly research-oriented faculty, limits to the 3–year MD—stem more or less from how the old answers cannot resolve new problems.

- [The problem is] reconciling a holistic view of medicine and medical practice with the need to master an increasingly complex basic science of medicine and especially molecular biology. In the MD program at McMaster we try to do far too much in far too little time, and this cripples our students. We have, as you know, a 3–year program. [I: What next?] Straight curriculum review that gives a more unified appearance to the curriculum. For 10 years, the individual units of the MD program have had their own way. By now, many of the problems [in tutorial] have become just a long table of contents. Then we will take up the matter of a 4–year curriculum. In the process, we may also rediscover our roots, inasmuch as our roots lie in innovation, not in dogma. From 1969 to 1981, we had a unit in the MD curriculum on basic biological mechanisms underlying medicine. With the curriculum reform in 1981, the unit disappeared. The current MD program chair feels that a physician must start with the biological mechanisms of medical science and that this is a big deficit in our program. [I: Do you agree?] Yes, I do. As a pedagogue, I know that some things are hard to learn, especially in the biological sciences. In such areas, you need good teaching and knowledgeable teachers. But at McMaster, with the nonexpert tutors, we utterly abandoned the idea of a teacher. As it turns out, only one biostatistician has conducted a tutorial in the last 2 years. An epidemiologist on our faculty calls my view the "myth of the expert tutor" in contrast to the prevailing idea here that the nonexpert tutor performs better. All but one of the studies that I have read, however, show that the expert tutor is better than the nonexpert.

- Within the faculty of health sciences, the problem is with the matrix system. The MD program is one of the horizontal levels in the matrix. As MD program chair, I have very little opportunity to sit down with those department chairs whose departments constitute the vertical levels of the matrix. It is a problem because they are the people who control the resources. They recruit the faculty and they allocate time and priorities. The MD program here has great flexibility and autonomy built into it. For example, the MD chair and unit planners are chosen without any regard to departmental or disciplinary backgrounds. In this way, the MD planners can avoid the hours-counting and similar activities of the department. But you accomplish change by enlisting people with time, energy, and mental work, and these people are always department oriented. On paper there are rewards for other activities, but in fact nondepartment-related activities are not at all visible to the department chairs. In the past the departments were distanced intentionally by the MD program in order, presumably, to preserve its nondepartmental nature. But the resources were more plentiful then. It is much less possible for the MD program now to stand apart from the departments. I do not know who said it, but, "The measure of a great civilization is not what you build but what you maintain." In the MD program at McMaster, we cannot run on automatic pilot any more. So much has changed in the meantime. There has been a molecular genetic revolution in biology. Our structures are changing. And the MD program here will be downsized from 100 to 90 students, in all probability. It is not official, but it is anticipated. The residency will be downsized, too, because of the new tie between undergraduate and residency enrollments. In the province, there will have to be a one-to-one ratio, 500 medical students to 500 residents each year. This really limits our long-term flexibility. Among other things, it makes it impossible for physicians to come back to retrain. Plus we are now going to 2–year licensure and therefore internships are effectively disappearing. With all this, you go into either family medicine or subspecialty residencies, period. Students thus have to make long-term decisions very early in their medical education. At McMaster this is an even greater problem for students, because we maintain a 3–year program.

- The major problem is ... whether to graduate MDs who are more public health oriented [or who are more] science oriented. At the program level this amounts to deciding what our product should be. For example, are students getting enough of the biological basis of medical education and practice? Are they getting enough quality in this area, and what is enough, anyway? In my view, they do not need more of the basic science disciplines separately, but they do need to be exposed to the emerging biological themes, [to the] emerging unity to the biological process as we study it and understand it. Being problem based, the program is centered around a clinical problem-solving method in which there is not enough conceptual content. [I: Can this be fixed?] Yes, absolutely, but people first have to agree that it is a problem and then work with the unit planners to build that agenda into the units. Our new chair of the MD program is just starting this. Another problem ... is related to program organization and to what we call the matrix system. The idea of vertical disciplines and horizontal programs was originally meant to separate resources from functions so as to bring appropriate resources together constructively around different functions. The problem has been that people holding the resources, the department chairs, are able to fry almost whatever fish they want [and] are too little accountable. What happens then is that individuals responsible for one function must enter a bazaar in which they must bid against other individuals responsible for other functions and thus it becomes a bidding war in which the chairs holding the resources may sell these according to their own interests. The competing buyers include MD program people, undergraduate science program people, graduate studies program people, and research program people. The system breaks down because the chairs decide, and these decisions may favor one program over another. So the constant issue through all these years is the problem with our matrix in distributing resources. The difference now is that there is an increasing will to do something about this problem. We are almost finished constructing a database on who is doing what in the MD program. This database will allow us to determine exactly what and how much people are contributing in the educational realm. Soon, therefore, the department chairs and the associate dean for education will be able to identify where resources for educational purposes are being underutilized, and this will help us create more accountability of the sort that I just described.

- [The problem is to restore] a consumer-driven . . . definition of medical education [and] student . . . awareness [of the need] for patient, rather than strictly physician decision making. [I: For whom are these the major problems at McMaster and for whom not?] It would be nonphysicians who would not agree with my definition . . . the PhD candidates, the people being trained in occupational and physical therapy, those being trained in administration, nurses and so forth . . . those who have been engendered into the traditional belief system, the kind that prevails at some of the British schools and at the University of Toronto. Traditionally trained MDs and the traditional MD program faculty rarely have a broad population viewpoint. They view the medical school as a trade school, a professional school, period. Also it would be the older group—those who have not yet recognized that the old sense of entitlement in being a physician no longer exists in the eyes of the public—that would not agree with my definition.

But McMaster problems also stem from the broader 1980s resource crunch and related research- and clinic-revenue imperative as much as any school in this study.

- Funding has become a major problem. The 1980s . . . were the years when the need first arose to earn your way right from the start as a faculty person here. In contrast, when I came to McMaster in 1969, my beginning salary was 90% base and 10% ceiling. By now, it is almost exactly the opposite. Thus the structure of salaries at McMaster has changed. The pressure on people to earn their way also comes from the fact that we have no big endowment here, no property and so forth, because we have not done any investing. The result of all this is that there are more cynics among us now. In recent years we have recruited to support research activity and this has brought in very unsympathetic and cynical attitudes to reforming the curriculum. Given the fact that we run on tutors and tutorials, this growing emphasis on research and on earning your own way here has meant that people like me must sustain workloads like mine. It is all quite demanding for most of us, and for too many this level of activity now depends on the guts and heart approach. It does not match well with research science. In fact, in some ways the research institute is antithetical to the matrix-managed system at McMaster. In the matrix, theoretically, each unit feels the tension of the other. It is like a tennis racket, inasmuch as if one string goes, the whole thing goes. In contrast, a research institute hives off from this sort of structure and is essentially an inward-looking sort of structure. [I: Had we spoken 8 to 10 years ago?] I would have said all of the above. In the 1983 revision . . . the truth is that we changed the curriculum as much around resource issues as anything else. People will say that we had a thoughtful review and so forth, but the original motivations for the changes in 1983 came from my phase 3 committee, and I know very well that it was a resource crunch, really, that produced the change.

In 1969, we started with 20 students. The class of 1972–1973 therefore had 20 students and it was wonderful. Then later 40 students was great and then 60 students was fine. But after 80 and up to 100 students, we definitely began to have resource problems. In the late 1970s, my committee was asked by the dean whether we could go to 100 students. We said, "No, we cannot," and we gave him the reasons. If you look at the curriculum as it was modified in 1983, it was designed to be divided by three. For example, with 75 students, there were three groups of 25 each, and all our resources were apportioned accordingly. With 100 students, the groups are divided into 33⅓, and the irony is that the changes that were brought into the curriculum in 1983 were intended to reduce the stress on tutors. Our original recommendations for curriculum change went through the MD committee and were adopted. They tried to make these changes educationally relevant but our recommendations were first and foremost tied to the resource demands of a 3–year curriculum with 100 students. The problem with a 3–year program is that there is no down time. It contains the same amount of material as 4 years. [I: Has anyone considered changing to 4 years?] We have talked about that for 25 years. [I: What is the reason why not?] Funding. At the start, the government wanted the efficiency of a 3–year program. The problem now is that it would increase the student body from 300 to 400 students. Thus it is discussed perennially but to date we have got only to an enrichment year, some of which is remedial and some of which is real enrichment. Only about 10% of our students take advantage of it. Then, too, our admission age is 3 to 4 years older than the norm in Ontario, and so our students tend to want a 3–year program. This diversity, after all, is what makes this school so exciting, and they want to get into the business of medicine sooner rather than later.

The problem at Sherbrooke, as at Hawaii, is to consolidate top-down change. Sherbrooke's troubles—strains on infrastructure, converting basic and clinical scientists to problem-based learning, practice-plan competition for faculty time, uneven teaching loads and unequal earning capacity, problem-writing for tutorials, depth of learning by students—are like McMaster's, more or less connected by a thread in this case the rigors of across-the-board change. Sherbrooke is a lab for how completely problems change when curriculum is transformed.

- The major problem . . . is in the 25% increase in our faculty, which itself is the result of hiring more people and having more students. The extension of activity has been a major stress for the University Hospital Center of

Sherbrooke . . . our teaching hospital. They have had great difficulty coping with the expansion of faculty. They have had to say to new faculty that we lacked infrastructure. The problem is based on the fact that the funding for the hospital comes from the Ministry of Health, whereas that for the university comes from the Ministry of Higher Education. In effect, we created an inflation problem in the hospital. We created more physicians, more services, and more growth than was expected.

- The real problem concerns resources. If you increase the amount of time that faculty are required to devote to students, you have to pay them for that, and we did not have new sources of money. Because of the change in our mission to problem-based learning, we have asked faculty for more time since 1985–1986, and from undergraduate faculty it has been possible to ask for this, especially in their role as tutors. But in changing the curriculum we have also changed the clinical skills unit. This now starts right in the first year. The difficulty has been to have the same degree of involvement on the clinical side, where teachers are called monitors, not tutors. The monitors have the same function as they have had for the past 10 to 20 years, but there has been a drastic change now in forms of communication and teaching. It is difficult to bring them into student-oriented teaching. We have been less successful in presenting the monitor as a new role consistent with our new mission. Thus, although on paper we have made major changes in the clerkship part of the undergraduate curriculum and extended it now over the entire 4 years, we still have in fact only half-realized this change. On the clerkship side, we did not sit down and plan strategy. We did not involve the clinical department directors as deeply as we did the preclinical department directors. We were just confident that people would follow. We were confident about this because of the great success that we had had in the first 2½ years, and we were likewise confident because a good half of the monitors were also tutors. But it proved more difficult than we thought, and it will take us longer to institutionalize these changes.
- For the basic scientists, before the new curriculum, teach-

ing was very stratified. There were 100 students in a lecture room and you just threw material at them. Basically you did not give a damn what the students came out with. It was a very convenient way to discharge your duties. It was the same here as it was in the European lecture system, and in fact many here come from Europe, especially in the basic sciences. On the clinical side, the problem is . . . that every hour spent with students is an hour off remuneration. Thus, teaching duties are harder for clinicians in a very practical sense of the term. The more a clinician teaches, the less he can buy a new car, for example. There is a direct financial impact. The more clinicians teach, the less money they make, or the greater their workload becomes. Either way, the quality of life suffers. Another major problem is the preparation of problems for the tutorials, the establishment of problems, in other words. . . . Ten years ago they were talking about closing this medical faculty. Then, the issue was how to stay alive. It was really a time of crisis.

- We have a unique way of setting earnings at Sherbrooke. The dean by himself or through a committee sets the earnings of all faculty. Thus we do not have individual negotiations over salary. Both university money and clinical money are put into the same pot and distributed in this fashion. Each person's share in this distribution takes into account individual teaching activity from the undergraduate to the postgraduate level. Thus if I want to earn my full salary, I need to teach 1,100 hours a year. To have a division fully credited, each member has to contribute these 1,100 hours. If you have 10 people in the internal medicine division, this means 10 times 1,100 hours, and if the division does less teaching, it gets less. You have to admit that this is a lot of teaching, considering that a 4–week unit as teacher involves about 70 hours or units of teaching. . . . A salary of $150,000 total, for example, might consist of $70,000 for 1,100 hours of teaching units and $80,000 from clinical work. If you can make more than $80,000 in clinical work, by our system, 50% of the surplus goes into the welfare system of the group practice, for example, to support sabbaticals or pregnancy leaves, and you keep the

other 50%. . . . If you are in a well-paid specialty, you will
be less interested in teaching, it appears. And if you are in
a less-well-paid specialty, for example, family practice, then
you are more interested in teaching, because you can earn
about the same teaching as you can in clinical practice.
Now, what is the effect of this on the teaching body? The effect is a discrimination of teachers on the basis of clinical
type. One unit equals about $70 per hour. If I am a cardiac
surgeon, in 1 hour I can earn much more than $70. Let us
say that I am planning a unit and want to pick some good
tutors. The cardiologist says no, obviously, so the students
do not have access to the cardiologist. The result is that
most teachers in medical schools are from departments of
pediatrics and departments of medicine. Before implementing the new curriculum, the major problem at the clinical
level would have been that clinical faculty did not have access to teaching students. The general internists and the
family practitioners rarely saw students, because everything was taught by subspecialists, from a very scientific
point of view with very little clinical and practical content
or concern.

- We are a small faculty and have to compete with the big
ones and so it is harder to attract faculty in some areas like
biogenetics to the University of Sherbrooke. [A related]
problem concerns our mission with respect to the population [of] the eastern township region in which we are located. This constitutes 8–10% of the Quebec population.
Therefore we have only about 8–10% of the power in these
matters [with only] about 410,000 people involved. Thus we
always have to spread out and we never have enough resources. When you need technical resources, you have to go
to the government and there you compete, for example,
with a super cardiologist at one of the larger schools. We
find this very difficult. In this light, what makes me very
happy about undergraduate medical education here at
Sherbrooke is that we can compete evenly with the big
schools in this field.

- What we teach, students do understand well, it appears, because they succeed in the exams. But I am afraid that there
are big holes in their knowledge of the fundamental sci-

ences, and I do not know if these are filled later or not. As a fundamentalist, there are things that you want students to know before they leave school. At present, we have no systematic way of knowing what they leave with. [The national boards] are not enough to ascertain whether students have adequate basic knowledge. I think, for example, that they should have more molecular biology, even though they will succeed in the external exam with very little knowledge of molecular biology. [I: Are there any measures, then, to ascertain whether there are holes in their knowledge?] A committee would be fine, composed of one person per unit, to review the materials being taught and to correlate them with the materials from other units. At present, we do not have the time to review these materials as a whole. . . . Under the old system, we began to realize that we were adding, adding, adding, never substituting material; that was the big problem. Each wanted more hours to teach. In those days, if you had told me that I could leave half the bacteriology out that I was teaching without any harm to the students, I would have just cried. Now I think it is quite okay.

Critics at Sherbrooke, as at Hawaii and New Mexico, do not hesitate to attribute the problems that they perceive—excessive teaching demands, neglect of research and professional activity, student discontent with the new pedagogy, the dogmatic mentality of reformers, a merely technical content of training—to the new curriculum.

- The main problem [is that] this way of teaching is quite heavy in terms of human resources [and] time is . . . inevitably taken away from research and professional activity. . . . The second problem [is that t]he human mind, I would say, is not that homogeneous, and this way of teaching that we now have is imposed on all students. I know that some would prefer another way of being taught. The attitude of the reformers here is a bit dogmatic. Because we are still recruiting the best students to Sherbrooke, however, it appears that teaching them one way or another will succeed despite itself. [I: Is the traditional system of teaching based on lectures better, in your view?] Yes. Either that or some combination of the different ways of teaching, as we were doing before. I think that some materials are best communicated in lecture and others in the application of knowledge within small groups. I believe that a combination of different teaching forms would be preferable to a single form. Our students ask for formal teaching once in a while, but it occurs this way only by student demand, when it occurs at all. And I have another disagreement with the current pedagogy. I think that it is not good to have a nonspecialist teacher dealing with a specialized subject.[I: Had we spoken 8 to 10 years ago?] The way we are teaching now comes from pressure from the public to produce physicians to take care of large populations. . . . The need for changing our curriculum came from this process over the last decade. When I first started teaching, the object here was the best scientific type of doctor, one trained to take care of all possible kinds of things, with a strong scientific background. Nowadays, we produce more technician types of physicians, people who always have to refer complicated problems to other people, even while there will be fewer and fewer of these latter. From the government's point of view, this is good policy because it is cheap medicine. Looking at the way things are going, with nurses increasingly knowledgeable and adding courses to their curriculum, in the next decade the nurses and the physicians that we train will be much the same, and this is good for the provincial government. [I: Is this a conscious motive on the part of the provincial government?] Yes. [I: Is there anything good about that motive?] No, not other than cost. It will produce cheap medicine, but it will be like medicine in the formerly communist countries.

The students are the same now as they have been [for the last] 25 years. They come in with no Latin, no Greek, no philosophy, and very little literature. I believe that to have a wide mind in the domain of medicine, you need Greek and Latin. It is not indispensable but it widens the mind. In anatomy or physiology, for example, our students do not have the very basic things, the bare minimum parts of the body, the place in evolution of our species. Now, with our new method they will not acquire them either during their medical education. [With the previous curriculum] they were exposed to some extent, because the professor would insert a few pearls into their reasoning. We had some really great teachers in the previous curriculum, but they were limited, in part, because of the type of students we had. With the raw materials that we have, namely, high intellectual caliber, low prerequisites, a short period of time, and the current method of problem-based learning, we do turn out remarkably good people for what the consumers need out there. But I think that we are depriving our students of their rights as human beings and as doctors. I think that we make superb technicians for the region, superb medical labor. But I ask myself whether this is the mission of a technical school or a medical school. I ask myself whether these will be the kinds of people I worked with at Barcelona, McGill, and Chicago. I admire what we have done here at Sherbrooke, but I am always aware also of what we are not doing. There is very little opportunity to teach the things you could teach before.

Supporters rightly worry about faculty burnout and related loss of momentum for the change.

- First, human resources here have been overutilized. There has been a lot of pressure on teachers due to problem-based learning. The workload for teachers is much heavier than 6 years ago. Resources are overutilized here. Fortunately, in the last 3 years, we have hired a lot of new people and this has helped. The second problem is that there is no change going on at Sherbrooke any more. All the problems were developed 3 years ago, when there was a lot of change. Now we are at risk simply to repeat and to regress. There is a risk of slowdown, of stasis now. People do not have the energy to improve all the time. We have been at it for 3 years now, people think, and we need a rest. [Ten years ago,] the main problem was stasis. There was far too much concern with results on the final exams. There was too much teacher-centered learning. We were always developing content and lecturing, whereas the students on their part were not involved and were passive spectators only. Therefore undergraduate education was not as important compared to postgraduate education or to research. The reform has increased the importance of undergraduate education and created more drive or zest in the faculty.

• The challenge of maintaining the reform, this is the big problem, how to reinject, modify, and improve recurrently. This will take a lot of resources, especially human resources. This is a small faculty, and human resources are limited. In the last 5 to 6 years, our process has taken a lot of energy. To maintain it will take a lot more. My fear is that our resources might not be enough to do this, [resulting in] stagnation from fatigue, both in the program's content and in its evaluation. I do not think it will happen, but this is the challenge.

CHAPTER 3

Faculty Morale

Faculty morale at Mercer, now in its second decade of operation, is down compared to the start-up years of purity and danger, especially among clinicians who bear the hospital's greater interest in earning revenue than in educating medical students.

- Relative to other schools that I know [morale] is somewhere between good to excellent. Relative to Mercer ... clinical faculty are lower at the moment because they have to deal with this hospital situation. The hospital administration emphasizes money and practice income only and de-emphasizes the education process. Our clinical faculty, therefore, live in two worlds, the medical education and residency world, in which all is going well, and the hospital medical center world, in which educational work is not valued. The medical center is really just a big community hospital where research is pooh-poohed, I guess. You just do not work happily in an institution that gives you these messages. As for basic-science faculty we have lost practically none of them. Only two or three have left on their own. [I: Had we spoken 10 years ago?] We all had the newness earlier on. There was a common enemy. There was a oneness of purpose that we all had. As chair here, I forbade something that I hated so much at Michigan State. I made it clear to everyone that I refused to believe in the second-class-citizens system. These were the teachers at Michigan State. I said that I would negotiate a person's time so that it might vary between teaching and other activities but that everyone was going to work a full day for full pay. I said that some may do only two tutorials but that those who did four tutorials would be just as valued and appreciated at Mercer as research lab people. I know that this attitude either comes or does not come from the administration of a medical school. And we pulled it off! Nobody at Mercer does zero in on one area. [I: Do you give career recognition for excellence in teaching?] Nobody is tenured in the basic sciences without publications. It is fine if some of the senior faculty have not published much, given all the time they spend working on school matters. But of course they are already tenured. For those not hired with tenure, even if they are reasonably good teachers, if they have no publications, they are not tenured. On the other hand, people who have made a fair effort at research, have a few publications, and do committee work, if they are also good teachers, we do give them tenure. So research does matter. But there are also people who were superb researchers but could not teach and they are gone. Education is extraordinarily important to us.

At Hawaii, as at Sherbrooke, the complete changeover to problem-based learning has vivified some but depressed others. Some faculty experience burnout and, especially among basic scientists, a loss of primary affiliation to the department.

- The problem is that there is wide variation [in morale]. It depends on how you feel about, whether you agree with the new curriculum. I would say that in the past 5 years I have never worked so hard in my life. I feel kind of burnt out. I think that I probably do not spend as much time in department affairs, for example, in just meeting with faculty. Leadership in the department has suffered.

If basic scientists at Hawaii feel dislodged by the actuality of change, their counterparts at New Mexico, shielded to date by the experiment's having been tracked onto a separate curriculum, are now agitated by the "best of both" primary-care and traditional-track unification that the school is initiating.

- Looking at change is uncomfortable. That is what is going on now nationally. Looking at change for people who have gotten into a kind of habit pattern makes them nervous. The preclinical people wonder whether they are still going to be able to do research, given the changes that we are undergoing in curriculum, while the clinical people see it in terms of teaching versus patient care balance. At the moment, there is no set schedule and the unknown is unsettling. . . . The premise that we are working on now is to combine the best of both the traditional and the primary-care curriculum, to merge them. The worst-case scenario is that the best of both are not identified organizationally. Medical students are very bright, and, almost independently of how you arrange things, they will learn. My experience is that there are some who are compulsive and want clear examinations and so forth and others who prefer a lighter structure and to do it themselves. I do not know what is going to happen to each of these groups by integrating the two curricula. It is an unknown and an experiment. There is no perfection. It is all yet to be seen. Fortunately, medical students will survive. [I: How do primary-care curriculum students affected perform on parts one and two of the national boards?] We have had students who have scored from the first to the ninety-ninth percentile on part one of the national boards, and, if we see a significant drop in scores on basic science A, B, or C in part one of the boards, then we go and talk to that particular chair. It is common knowledge with chairs, moreover, that the primary care curriculum students do not score as high on part one of the national boards as traditional-track students but do score a little better on part two. We are not quite sure how to interpret this. In both tracks, however, the best students on part one continue to be the best on part two.
- I am the wrong person to ask. I am a cock-eyed optimist. People I interact with are pretty good, I would say, although there are some problems. People say that they are asked to do too much here without enough support. But I think it is the busy people who have the good morale. It is the productive faculty who feel unburdened and who are willing to teach in both the primary-care and traditional

tracks. Not a lot of people are jumping ship. Some of the basic scientists find it harder to get grants and are still pres-
sured by the dean to bring in grant money. Still we have
many faculty in the planning process, and it is the minority who think that the primary-care-curriculum clique is
shoving things down their throat. If we just converted in total to the primary-care curriculum, it would be much easier. Instead, we are trying to integrate the new curriculum
and the traditional approach.

Morale at mainstream Minnesota is good. The place is
abustle and a new research complex has just opened. Still, some
faculty are daunted, as they might be when faculty salaries so
depend on outside funds, by drops in NIH (National Institutes of
Health) and other research support. Too, the "assault" from a
very competitive health care environment, which threatens the
school's patient base, causes deep concern.

- [Morale is] very good, although there is some concern about
  the school's ability to contend with the vicissitudes of the
  moment and be effective on all three legs of the mission
  stool. Then too, there is some concern among younger clinical faculty with respect to research support and their ful-
  fillment of patient-care expectations. And there is general
  concern about the magnitude of competition for NIH funding, which has been dropping in recent years. Some are
  down-spirited about that. [I: Is there any sense of renewal
  with respect to the undergraduate curriculum?] That depends on whom you talk to. There are a lot of people who
  are heavily involved in the new emphasis on primary care.
  And, with several new and exciting initiatives in research
  here, there is a lot of networking going on too. In neuroscience, beginning 8 years ago, there has been a large recruitment across several departments, which together have
  developed a very successful research and graduate program. There is a comparable interdepartmental effort in
  human genetics, which is founded on molecular biology
  and molecular structure. In biomedical engineering, there
  is a strong research program at the physics–biology interface. There is the Cancer Center focus, and developmental

biology is very active here. What I most fear is an assembly-line view of medicine and medical education. In this view, you define the outcome as a limited degree of performance expectation and then you design the assembly line to produce just that. The problem is that that level of performance will be unable to cope with change in medicine. Above all, products of that assembly line will be unable to exercise independent judgment. For me, this is the purpose of exposing medical students to research. It is so that they will learn intellectual inquiry, that they will understand how to ask questions, not just to parrot answers.

• I would say that we have more of a siege mentality now because of a number of assaults from outside that have disturbed the groves. First, there is reduction in state support. (For the biennium 1991–1993, the university went to the state to request tens of millions of dollars to do various things, but it also said that it would be reducing enrollments at the same time. That was a big mistake, because the legislature looks first of all at enrollments and said, "Well, fewer students means less money." So the university was cut. Thus, in the year 1991–1992, there were no pay increases for university people anywhere. This included the medical school, which is viewed on campus as a fat cat even though we are earning money.) Second, there is the severe competition for medical care in the state, about which there is no end of newspaper articles. Third, there is a climate in medical practice in town that is not good. I mean that there is a town-gown rift, a rift between those physicians downtown and those up here. Fourth, there is a growing disaffection of our affiliated hospitals with our clinical faculty. The hospitals are facing strong competition problems. But there is no feeling of corporateness in the big departments of medicine. [I: If we had been speaking 10 years ago?] Then I would have thought that faculty morale was about as good as ever. There was a sense of corporate responsibility. Basic science heads got together to change the curriculum. People voted ballots, there were retreats, there was discussion.

At Case Western Reserve, morale is good among research-oriented faculty who, like their counterparts at Minnesota, have recently seen a new research tower completed. But to veterans of previous-cycle innovations, which created a net division of labor between department chairs' coordination of research and patient care and subject-committee chairs' coordination of curriculum, the present period is educationally uninteresting, even discouraging.

- [Morale is] relatively good. There are particular issues floating around, for example, the financial issue with the university. The university has allocated costs, and there are new charges now for utilities and for library services. A few months ago, there was a tremendous citywide effort focused on the medical school. The Cleveland Foundation people participated, along with other community and outside people. Ultimately, 6 months later faculty feel that very little has happened. They expected a lot of community financial support and, while there appears to be some, it is not of the magnitude that they anticipated. [I: If we had been speaking 5 years ago, would you have described faculty morale in similar or different terms?] About the same. Then the issue was that of research space. Some felt then that the school was not going anywhere. [I: And the new building helped that?] Yes, it helped a lot, along with the recruitment of new basic-science chairs. We found that we were missing critical elements in the new sciences, particularly genetics and molecular biology. [I: And in more recent years?] Now it is more that expectations are very high and people are asking, "Now where is the golden era?"
- In the 1950s, I was in transition from the department of biochemistry and basic science to the department of medicine. The department of biochemistry was feverish in its intensity. Harlan ran biochemistry as a democracy. Utter was his successor and his widow once told me that when Utter became chairman he hated, for example, to put forward his salary increase. At the time, the department of medicine was starting up and Rammel Kamp was head of preventive medicine. Kamp was spectacular and just full of ideas. It was exciting! There was a lot of good work being done. The administrators played an important role in all this but the educational process was governed by the gen-

eral faculty. Policy was set by the general faculty with input predominantly from the committee on medical education. Administration was by the dean of education down through the coordinator to the subject-committee chairs to the individual teachers. The coordinator picked subject-committee chairs who then went to the department chairs to arrange the curriculum. The subject-committee chairs had some real authority. [I: And now?] The separation of powers between department chairs who ran the departments and coordinated research efforts or patient care, on the one hand, and subject-committee chairs and teachers who were responsible for the curriculum, on the other, has largely disappeared. The current chair of the committee on medical education now turns directly to the department chairs to ask, "Who can I get to teach subject X, Y, or Z?" And often as not, the department chair will give you the guy who is least important to him rather than the best at teaching.

At Dartmouth, where within recent memory only a 2–year basic-science course of studies was offered, the prospect of changing its now very traditional 4–year curriculum has accentuated long-standing divisions, in the midst of Dartmouth's own financial crunch, between faculty and administration and between basic scientists and clinicians.

- The word that comes to mind is anxious. [I: About?] Change. I think that there is a group of basic scientists who are happy to see us bailed out but who hate our dependence on clinical dollars. The anxiety is about the way the problem was solved. They think that we are selling out to the clinical world. On the other hand, there are some clinical faculty who feel that I have done this in order to extract money from them. They are mad and anxious about their clinical dollars being threatened by coming political changes. For the most part, the teaching faculty is anxious about changing the curriculum. They are not sure that what is coming will be better, and they wonder whether it will take more of their time. I came at a funny time, after all. In 1988–1989 the institution did not seem to have a sense of itself. It was adrift. Its only purpose had been to complete the building, a $218 million project. When I came it was done and people were asking, What next?

We have been going through a medical-center-wide strategic planning process. The strategy planning committee is composed of me as head as well as the heads of the hospital, the clinic, the Thornton Health Center, and the V.A. The final statement will be issued April 1st. We have identified six strategies, the first of which is educational. The remaining five have to do with patient care, research, management and governance, information systems, and internal regulation systems. The educational part is composed of the New Directions Committee work, the Koop Institute, and the Robert Wood Johnson Generalists Initiative. The plan recently went out to all faculty for feedback and for discussion. This happened in November and December. There were 13 separate evening department meetings in this regard. I have either gotten the message from or met with every departmental member. Therefore, despite all the anxiety, at least we have a direction that we did not have before.

- [Morale is] low. Faculty feel under substantial financial pressure for maintaining research or clinical productivity. They also often feel that they are not adequately supported by the institution, that they are contributing their life blood to the place without a sense of adequate appreciation. This comes out of a recent period of financial restructuring and all the apprehension that goes with it. Our new dean has a different style of leadership, which has been essential from a structural point of view in a time of fiscal crisis and negative relations with the hospital and the clinic. But the way he is leading us out of these problems has cost considerably in faculty morale. This relates to the lack of a forum at Dartmouth in which we can talk, a lack of a sense of community. This is not entirely missing here, but we are limping along at best. For the last 20 years, this medical school has functioned like a very strong mom-and-pop grocery store. Wallace is trying to move it into a more sophisticated control system. Before, the medical school administration was benign but strongly ineffective. Now, it is

regarded as increasingly effective but considerably less caring.

- [Morale is] not terrific. The question is, are faculty members being squeezed to be more productive in research or in
  patient care at a time when new directions are emerging in
  the curriculum that would be more time demanding? The
  faculty at Dartmouth are already working 110%. Faculty
  tend to kind of deny the problem, hope it will go away. [I:
  What does this denial bode?] That the changes will be very
  difficult to make and to maintain without, first, an influx
  of big money and, second, personnel whose major or sole
  purpose is education.

At Harvard, the tone is guardedly optimistic, though morale among ambulatory-care instructors is reportedly undercut
by feelings of relative deprivation—receiving too little recognition for too much work—and by questions concerning whether
the new teacher–clinician track will truly meet their needs and
career goals. There are also rifts across reform currents themselves, especially between behavioral/primary-care-oriented and
more social/population-oriented faculty in particular, committed
as each is to broadening the school's dominant biomedical
model.

- Here there is tremendous value put on molecular biology.
  A problem that can be reduced to molecules is given the
  highest press. Basic science on campus is more and more
  driven by other forces than clinical needs, by its own fasci-
  nation in that it gives an incredible sense of power. This
  limits you to asking certain questions. If all research
  grants go to molecular biology then the other pieces of basic science are neglected, questions about cells and tissues,
  the rate of transfer of sugar across the rabbit ilium for example, [or about] the biopsychosocial. Today these other
  branches are not considered reduced enough by the molecular biologists.
- We have adopted ambulatory-care education by a variety of
  ways, in clerkships, in the patient–doctor course, and in
  electives. This creates a greater demand for primary-care
  physician-teachers, especially in the patient–doctor course,

[and] we have really had to look everywhere for these people. We contracted with the HCHP [Harvard Community Health Pla]] to pull off the clerkship in ambulatory care. There was a big discussion in the curriculum committee. Where on earth would the students find the clerkships? people asked. Our teaching hospitals did not have enough capacity for 160 students in ambulatory clerkships. Then there was the problem of rewarding these clinician–teachers so that they feel recognized by the medical school. They really felt left out, really unrecognized. So Dean Tosteson pushed faculty to create the clinician–teacher track and got [President] Bok to approve it. The downside is that younger potential faculty in the clinician-teacher track do not yet feel that it is real, that they will actually be promoted for their teaching. There is a lot of skepticism among these faculty, who are mostly instructors or assistants without tenure. [I: So the problem is to deliver on the promise of the new track?] Yes. We have asked primary care faculty to deliver for 8 years by now, by holding out a carrot. Now, there is a mounting problem of burnout. Some are not willing to do it anymore for Harvard, for the cause. I am worried about that. The dean believes that the new organization of students in societies will improve conditions for these faculty, that it will bring clinical faculty into the societies, that it will give them a forum, a home base. [I: Is he right?] Yes, but it is all happening at the same time, both new organization and real burnout. Many do not see how the new organization will improve matters. They do not see how the clinician–teacher track will address their problems. Maybe in 2 or 3 years time, but burnout for some is right now. Then, with burnout, students see no joy either in their primary-care physician teachers or in their encounters with patients. The predominant role model at Harvard after all is the researcher, and the predominant message [is] to get into specialty medicine.

Primary care faculty need academic role models too, instead of seeing that primary care and academic medicine are mutually exclusive. They need to feel heard and wanted. Faculty at places like HCHP have to feel part of the academic community. Until now, they have felt like second-class citizens. Their sense is that if you are not at a big teaching hospital, then you are not part of the community. We need to make them part of planning committees, part of course design groups, part of course leadership, for example, in the patient–doctor course. It is a vicious cycle really. You are in the clinician–teacher track at the instructor level, and then the dean says that course leaders must be full professors.

- One thing is to interdigitate clinical and basic-science experience more extensively and even to give students a year of clinical work before the basic sciences. Obviously this would have to be well supervised. As it is they have to be at the beginning of the third year to start clinical work. Starting at the first year might be more useful, on the first day, really. They might not have the science underpinning . . . but it could stimulate investing in these underpinnings. Then, in the second year of courses, they could see the relevance, feel the need to do the biosciences. [I: Is there any chance of this here?] Nope. First, it would be too threatening to the basic scientists. They could not primp the clinical people with the pathophysiology of the disease. Second, it would cost the clinical people too much time in their own perception.

- If you read *The New York Times Magazine* piece or watched the PBS [Public Broadcasting System] show on the New Pathway at Harvard, you would think that there had been a major change here. For example, you would think that there had been a dramatic increase in the social sciences in the curriculum and that its major goal was to make more humane doctors. Also if you read President Bok's statement on medical education, you would think that the population-based sciences, concepts and principles from the social sciences and humanities, were the primary goal of the curriculum reform here. I would say that this has not been it at all. In the first 2 years of the reform here, from 1985 to 1987, there was an increasing amount of time spent in some of these areas. Before the New Pathway, in the classical curriculum, students were required to select from a set of elective courses in a number of departments, which included social medicine, psychiatry, and preventive medicine. After, there was the patient–doctor course, planned and implemented largely by [a psychiatrist and an internist] around this content. Members of the department of social medicine did not participate much in this. People were still required to do some electives in social science, plus there was the entire block of 10 weeks devoted to the human life cycle, in which developmental issues are raised from birth to death. Soon, however, this content became the target of a number of forces and was virtually dismantled at Harvard. [I: Which forces?] Some basic scientists, for example. Their attitude was, "We have lost and you have gained." They prevailed on the curriculum committee. Thus the life-cycle course was lost and the basic scientists grabbed that time back. There was a lot of politicking . . . deals were cut and the time given to the social sciences in the medical curriculum reduced more and more. In the dismantling, however, the real problem was with the organization of the patient–doctor course. The split we got into was between tutorials, conducted by psychiatrists primarily, and lecture time, given to the social medicine department. These two points of view are very different. The split meant that the course was not very popular and, therefore, became vulnerable. What evolved out of this was a patient–doctor course in year 1 only and only for 2 hours every other week. In other words, the course was vastly watered down.

It has become, in large part, a course given by clinicians teaching medical students to talk to patients. It is no longer a serious joining of social science and clinical medicine. The course is now very superficial. The second year of the patient–doctor course has now been handed over to the old Introduction to Clinical Medicine course people, for whom there is absolutely no pretense of integrating relevant social science content. The second year is now completely out of the hands of any sort of social science people. The third year content in the patient–doctor course has been completely dismantled. The demise of the patient–doctor course is the demise of population-based content in the New Pathway curriculum, the demise of the portal through which this content could be introduced. The patient–doctor course was never really a patient–doctor–society course anyway. It was always just patient–doctor and reflected the unwillingness on the part of the medical school to build a serious population or community base into the curriculum change here. Even the Kaiser Foundation people in the mid-1980s supported preventative medicine only from the point of view of behavioral psychology, only in terms of individual behavior. Thus the population component has never really happened here.

- There is some hope in recent efforts people are dreaming up in the Holmes Society [whose] director has been mandated to organize activities around race, culture, ethnicity, and gender. We want to put students in places where they will not just be the physician but where they will have to relate to community people, where they are not the only authority. As it is, the surrounding community is not seen as a laboratory at the medical school, and most students spend 4 years without even crossing the street. They are in detached laboratory research for 4 years, and there is little research on populations. Those who are the radicals here are saying that students should spend more time in primary care, for example, at the Harvard Community Health Plan. Frankly, however, I think that American primary care is no more population-oriented than tertiary care is. In neither approach is there an investment in or development of an appropriate response to communities or to populations. Primary-care medicine, in my view, simply mirrors the structure of American health care in general. But one could imagine a curriculum that did things differently. For example, you might teach toxicology by studying the distribution of toxic substances in a community.

Morale at UCSF, a public school like Minnesota that has earned a reputation for excellence, is by nature upbeat but similarly undercut not so much by the forces or effects of internal transformation, educational or otherwise, as by reductions in the external support on which it so much depends.

- Until the last year or two [morale was] as good as you could find. [There was] a strong sense of belonging to a first-rate institution. We have a splendid dean who came 3½ year ago. He is very highly considered. But in the last year, especially, faculty have become deeply concerned about state support. We have lost one or two of our basic scientists for this reason. People feel that it has reached crisis proportions. The dean and the chancellor are meeting with the regents next week to discuss the problem. I do not think, however, that it has affected medical education as much as the research enterprise. The whole biotechnology industry spun out of here after all. But I am an optimist. I have been through many micro-crises. The school is phoenix-like. We have a shot at the Letterman Hospital and the Army Hospital at the Presidio . . . and we are looking for a new university chancellor. [I: Is leadership, university leadership important to you?] Extraordinarily important. [I: Is the dean or the chancellor more important?] It is the chancellor, not the dean, who deals with the regents. That said, we are doing very well at the micro-level. Students have excellent morale. And the recent graduates, 97 to 98% of them made donations to the school last year! This would not have happened 10–15 years ago.

- It is similar to morale at other medical schools. Everyone is concerned. NIH grants are way down. But here, space is an additional problem. The basic scientists feel the crunch in terms of fewer research dollars and the clinicians feel it because you can only do so many procedures per hour. It is hard for them to make the bucks of private practitioners. Therefore in terms of faculty morale, we were happier in the 1980s, in the times of boom or bust. It has been much tighter in the last couple of years.

Morale at the two Canadian schools differs considerably, given where each stands in the innovation process. At McMaster, public mission-bound like UCSF and Minnesota, it is dampened by reductions in outside support, both fiscal and societal, and by internal inhibitors that, ironically, have come with success and growth.

- Undermining morale now is the fact that people do not have the same enthusiasm that they once had about the McMaster way. The practice plan business was designed in order to alter the pay mechanism for faculty and to give them more money. [I: Did it work?] No! We work more now and have less time to think about what we are doing. Another thing that has changed us at McMaster is that the center of gravity has shifted from this institution to the other clinical teaching centers outside this building. This has come from the major financial pressures and cutbacks in the number of beds and has led to a significant faculty morale problem as the center has shifted to teaching hospitals such as the Hamilton Civic Hospital. These institutions have grown and developed much faster than this hospital. This has created real morale problems.

- [Morale] is lower than it should be. First, lack of [faculty] accountability results in big differentials in staffing the MD program. Second, there is the perception that contributions of the faculty to the educational process are not valued in terms of tenure and promotion. Everyone is feeling done in. We have reached a crossroads where the right for faculty to decide how to fulfill the social contract is being challenged at every level of society. This challenges the professional role of medical faculty. Faculty have not come to terms with how fundamental this change in society is. It is social and political, far from philosophical. It is horse-trading, not just speculation in ideas. The majority of faculty just do not feel appreciated anymore. [I: Had we been speaking 10 years ago?] It was a bit better then because the societal pressures were only just mounting then. Our reliance on the practice plan, on fee-for-service, to fund individual faculty was not as great then as it is now because we were just doing less then. The data show that at almost every medical school fee-for-service medicine has increased sharply as a proportion of total income at the same time that the number of students has remained virtually constant. [I: What is going on?] We have co-opted faculty practice plan money so as to pay more faculty to do more things. We are a victim of our own bullishness. We cannot blame government. Increasing fee-for-service income derived from the faculty practice plan and using these revenues to expand long-term care has been a good thing. Much has been accomplished. But the problem that comes with the success is a certain demoralization of awfully busy faculty and a certain devaluation of the education process.

- [Morale] is lower than it has ever been [because] of the decline here of the McMaster vision that we are unique, interesting, world-shattering, and that sort of thing, that we are part of a collective team working for a similar goal. This feeling is no longer as strong as it once was. It is going in the MD program and, in the broader faculty, it is going fast, especially in the big clinical departments like medicine and surgery and in the big billers, the big subspecialties. I have to say that it has gone too, to some degree, from the dean's office. It is the loss of shared vision and cohesiveness. This has occurred also because of our change in size from a faculty that started at less than a hundred. You cannot grow to over a thousand and agree on much of anything. [I: Had we been speaking 10 years ago?] Then, the climate would have been less vehement, more accepting, less strong, less obsessive. I would say that now we do not have much of a moderate, middle-of-the-road section of the faculty here, with a "let us try things" stance anymore.

- The profession of medicine is demoralized and we have personalized it as our own fault, the fault of the program. I hear faculty, sitting around between calls, converse about medicine. They say that it is not what it used to be and that they would not enter it again under present circumstances. And this gets communicated to students. Education is in fact a lot like parenting. Why send others into medicine when you are demoralized yourself? I would ask. In clinical care delivery, time is increasingly department-regulated and restricted. There are big cutbacks in operating rooms as well as in hospital beds and resident slots. It is also much harder to get grants. Our faculty has not been rewarded for doing good things in the province, moreover. We reorganized to be more efficient in health care delivery but then were hit with the same freeze as every other region in Ontario. So there really is no incentive to be more efficient.

- [Morale] is better than it was a year ago, when the MD committee was a small debating society, a mafia that spoke in tongues. Outside that committee was a large and disaffected faculty that is smart and has a lot of common sense. These were largely disenfranchised with respect to making decisions about teaching and content. It was harder and harder to get tutors for the MD problems. Opposition was passive and sullen and there was a sense that most people did not give a good damn about the program. With the new MD committee, the rank and file have taken over again. [I: With what result?] We have not changed at all in a decade and now all sorts of things are possible. There has been a steady decline in morale from 1982 until last year. Since then morale had risen sharply. Ten years ago, before the decline set in, we were still the new boys on the block, like the University of New Mexico 5 years ago, and we were still going around the world proselytizing. [I: What was it that brought on the change in morale?] The whole program became routine. We became like middle-aged churchgoers reciting the old songs but wondering why we were doing it anymore.

- [Morale] is picking up now [compared to] 1987–1991 [when] we were hanging on by a thread and many people were very demoralized. [In these years] people would put up grand schemes but never stick around to do the homesteading. It was all just endless talk. One of the really vital things, nevertheless, about the tutorial system is that you learn to identify things that you do not know and come clean about them. This is what we have recently done in the MD program and this is why things are picking up now. So morale is much improved, anxious but good. Faculty are anxious because of various outside forces. Because of the need to bill, they ask, "How the hell am I going to do the other stuff required of me here when I do 25 to 30 hours of patient care a week?" But there is now a push inside the program to give a lot of support and recognition, to tell faculty that the educational part of the MD program is very important. Even so, many find that it is a nightmare trying to fit in all the tasks that they have to perform in the program, and I personally wonder how much longer people will be prepared to lead these crazy lives at half the salary that they could earn in private practice. [I: Ten years ago?]

We were paralyzed. The then-chair of the MD program was in a constant fight with the dean.

At Sherbrooke, finally, morale is not bad, despite how taxing the new curriculum has been for many. Most agree that the changeover did save the school, which no longer fears for its survival. Students appear to be performing as well or better than before on boards. And instead of faculty retrenchment there has been hiring, albeit too much of it from within.

- Everybody is working very hard. Demands are high in teaching, research, and clinics. People here work at a very high level, but morale is good. If we look at each part of the new curriculum, the committees are still very active.
- They are proud of what we have done, but they are also tired. The amount of time and work involved in student–teacher contact. The lecture system required far less time. You had one teacher and 60 students. Now with the tutorial system, you have six teachers with 10 students each and two tutorials and two preparations a week. This is why we have had to hire new teachers, to share out the activities, including clinical activities, to share out the whole load. [I: Ten years ago?] Before the change here, faculty were depressed. We were not proud of what we were doing. We were negative, sarcastic, and cynical. It may be that we will arrive back at this in 5 or 10 years if we become static again. Therefore curriculum renewal must be an ongoing process. It cannot be a wholesale, major renewal as before, but it must be ongoing.
- [Morale] is pretty good . . . I think [because of] the group practice plan. People stay here because they like it. It is organized in such a way that you can earn enough as long as your expectations are not too grand, for example, to have a big house or drive a Mercedes. You are guaranteed reasonable earnings, a decent office, the opportunity to find partners in your practice, and good colleagues. Planning here facilitates groups of individuals who are committed to common goals in teaching, research, or patient care. It is easy to communicate here. There is a lot of talk in the halls.

When the new curriculum started, people thought that they would have no time to do research or to teach residents; there was a lot of talk against the program. However, with time and experience in tutorials, most have discovered that they enjoy doing these things. There is now less self-pity, less irony, less criticism and so forth. Now people are doing more tutorials than before, and largely voluntarily. [I: Has the new curriculum become legitimate?] Yes. [I: Since when?] Really in the last 2 years. Before, people were worrying that students did not know as much, because they were not getting lectures. They thought that there would be problems with the national exams. They thought that there would be problems when they got to clinics. But all these worries were addressed by experience, and we have discovered that our students now may not be better, but they are not worse in all these respects, including the national exams. Thus, the major worries have been invalidated by experience. Ten years ago was a very bad period. There were major cutbacks in university positions. It came from the government, which said to medical school graduates, "If you do not go to university hospitals and you end up in a private practice in a major city, then you will get to keep only 70% of your fees for medical services provided patients under the national plan." So the government really motivated us to stay in the university and it helped the university become more competitive with private practice. We started recruiting young people, we developed an endowment system from the practice plan, and in part this has functioned as a fund to send residents to places like the Mayo Clinic. There are now five of us in the department and three have taken advantage of such residencies, for example, at the Institute of Neurology in London, Queen's Square, at the Mayo Clinic, and at the University of Western Ontario in London. In this way we started having the means to attract and train people better. The faculty practice plan and its endowment, therefore, has been a great help for faculty morale. It has provided fresh input. [I: How established has the practice of internal recruitment become?] Initially, with our first graduates between 1969–1972, there was a high degree of internal re-

cruitment. After that, there was a decline of internal
recruitment and inbreeding and very few came in this way
in the years from 1979–1985. The second wave of such recruitment occurred following the year 1986. Typical of this
period is that a person earns his/her MD and then does his/
her residency here, then takes a 2–year fellowship with our
money to go to another place.

- The people I know are fine. In fact, I would say it is better
  and better each year. At first many were opposed to the
  new curriculum, many were very frustrated. Now it is
  fewer and fewer. I would say that the vast majority are
  quite happy and that most do not regret the change at all.
  [I: What is the primary thing that people like about the
  new curriculum?] It is the contact with students and discussion as opposed to long lectures in big arenas. [I: If we
  had been speaking 6 or 8 years ago?] Most people were very
  afraid to change 6 years ago. There was a lot of fear, of
  course. [I: What were they afraid of?] It was not really of
  losing their jobs, as much as of losing power, maybe. Most
  were professors who were teaching 30 or 40 hours a year
  and who were in control of the material. When they realized that they were no longer in control of the material,
  that they had very little control in fact, they did not like
  that idea at all. Another thing that they were afraid of was
  the time. At the start we had no idea how much time would
  be involved, but we soon learned.

As at Hawaii and New Mexico and, again, especially
among basic scientists who feel disempowered by problem-based
learning, some at Sherbrooke remain ambivalent.

- [Morale is] bad. My feeling is that the majority of teachers
  do not agree with this way of teaching. But within this distribution of views there is a large standard deviation. I
  would add that average morale is probably positive because
  the enthusiasts here are very enthusiastic. [I: Is disagreement based in any particular areas?] Among the basic scientists the feeling is stronger than among the clinicians. I
  may be wrong, but I think that the way we used to teach,
  by formal lecture, was a quite demanding way to teach in

terms of preparation time, to name only one aspect. I think that it was more demanding than the new curriculum, where instruction is much more passive. For many natural scientists, it is now easier to teach and less challenging. Maybe there is another factor, too. In the old system, I had the feeling that there were only a few very good professors, even though at Sherbrooke everyone in principle has to teach. I think that those who were not good teachers felt bad, since they had to teach. So instead of improving themselves, they decided to change the whole way of teaching as a way to deal with the problem. The evidence for my statement here is that teachers whom students like the most are not those who have promoted problem-based learning. Those who have promoted the new curriculum were not the best teachers before. [I: If we had been speaking 10 years ago?] Better, more enthusiastic across-the-board. But in the early 1980s it began to change for the worse, because of money, resources, and facilities. It had to do with the broader economic cycle in the province and in the country and in effects of this on research support and so forth.

P<small>ART</small> 2

Innovation Process

To investigate how the 10 schools under study have actually gone about changing their education programs and, among schools, how similar or different the process by which they innovated may have been, in part 2 we shall compare and contrast characterizations of change impetus, design, and implementation. Proceeding stepwise through the change process, we shall also look at how the process may vary school by school according to sponsorship (more administration-driven or faculty-based), scope (more across-the-board or within-bounds), and consequence (more person-dependent or more institution-embodied, hence more or less lasting in effect). As in part 1, certain defining characteristics—public–private, older–younger, earlier–later innovator status, as well as school size—will be examined for how they give warp to the weave, here of change process.

In chapter 4, we will see that in change impetus and sponsorship there are patterns. Readers may recall that phrases, used throughout part 2 of this volume, such as innovating "down a column" and "across a row," derive their meaning from the program and curriculum tables often presented in medical school catalogues in which horizontal rows depict program years and vertical columns show separate programs or tracks. Innovating "across a row," therefore, might involve changing first-year teaching methods or putting second-year material together in a new way; "across several rows," integrating previously separate first- and second-year material; "down a column," establishing an entirely new pathway or program of studies down through 2, 3, or 4 years. Innovating "across-the-board," in contrast, means redesigning rows and columns altogether. Thus at Hawaii, Sherbrooke, New Mexico, and Minne-

sota, innovation of quite different scope, across-the-board in the
former cases, down an experimental column at the third, and
across a row at the last, is prompted by individuals acting from
quite personal visions and charisma. These include, respectively, a clinical faculty member becoming dean who had long
bided his time, a dean-supported administrator brought in from
outside, a pair of inventor–faculty, and a medical ethicist-basic
scientist team. Dartmouth's specific effort to put clerkships in
outpatient settings is likewise the *vox clamantis in deserto* of a
single individual.

At Harvard, UCSF, Mercer, and McMaster in contrast, impetus for equally diverse sorts of innovation—down one column
at the former, across rows at the latter three—is prompted more
nearly by institutions acting on quite corporate visions through
individuals. Not to deny personal agency, individuals at these
schools profess to act more from institutional legacy than from
personal vision, legacies, respectively, of having long been excellent at everything, recently become excellent at many things,
recently become excellent at one thing, and long been distinc-
tively different. The current conversations about innovation at
Case Western Reserve and Dartmouth likewise derive more
from institutional than individual charisma, in the former's rec-
ollection that it once profoundly innovated and the latter's felt
need as a 4–year program to keep the distinguished company
that it had as a 2–year medical school.

The fact that Hawaii, Sherbrooke, New Mexico, and Minnesota are all public and, in three of four cases, smaller and younger suggests that—at whatever level they may have innovated—
individuals at these schools have more latitude than at the
others to bend the institution to their own visions. Harvard,
UCSF, and McMaster suggest the obverse, that eminence, re-
mote or recent, spills over into innovation efforts, setting high
standards but also bending personal vision to institutional legacy. Part of big, high-status academic health centers in which
medical education consumes only a fraction of overall expenditures, the former two medical schools would probably not, without decanal leadership, have made innovating in predoctoral instruction, which is an end in itself.

Chapter 4 will reveal that the top administrator either
sponsors change, as at Mercer, Hawaii, Sherbrooke, Harvard,

and UCSF, or otherwise fosters it, as at New Mexico and Mc-Master, so much so that the critical importance of such sponsorship cannot be questioned. Where it is less in evidence, as at Dartmouth, Minnesota, and Case Western Reserve, and initiative is left more to lower administrators or to faculty, change may be no less original, but it is usually more circumscribed.

In chapter 5, a pattern will emerge in the scope of change that is designed at these 10 schools. Schools that design broader-scope, across-the-board change, including Mercer, Hawaii, Sherbrooke, and now New Mexico, are for the most part younger, smaller, public (Mercer is one-third state supported), and more mission-distinct. Those who design narrower-scope, within-bounds change—down a column at Harvard, across several rows at UCSF and McMaster, across one row at Minnesota, Dartmouth, and (though more in research and service than in teaching) Case Western Reserve—are not so much private as older, larger, and more mission-comprehensive medical schools located in big academic health centers. Thus the larger the school, the narrower the scope of change may be at private and public institutions alike.

In chapter 6, we will witness a range of implementation efforts, some conducted more by administrators, senior or junior, as at Hawaii, New Mexico, and Dartmouth; some more by individual faculty members, as at Minnesota; some more by administrator–faculty combinations, as at Mercer, Harvard, UCSF, McMaster, and Sherbrooke. If the latter, combined effort is observed at every sort of school, the administrator-led effort appears more characteristic of the smaller, more easily orchestrated schools, and the faculty-led effort more characteristic of the two earlier cycle innovators, Minnesota and Case Western Reserve, where recent research- and clinic-revenue-compelled administrations have put education reform legacies largely in the past tense.

As for the consequences related in chapter 7, the combined administration–faculty efforts depend less on one fearless individual as time goes on and thus permit a higher degree of institutionalization. Pegging change of any scope on the leadership of one or a few—a dean at Hawaii, an administrator at Dartmouth, one or two faculty members at Minnesota—is risky for lasting effects, given the many ways that individuals may fall away.

Several findings will criss-cross the four chapters that follow. Foremost is that disciplinary-department-based organization—in how it distributes resources, creates and transmits knowledge, and rewards faculty—is usually not very receptive to schoolwide or programwide current-cycle curriculum reform efforts. Basic scientists especially, still the core faculty to most predoctoral curricula, do not readily accept these efforts, because they are the ones who have most to modify how and what they teach in the process. Clinical faculty may have less to modify and to lose, thus be more receptive to change, though too few of the schools studied here have innovated as profoundly in clinical instruction to gauge whether this is so.

But it will also emerge that deans appointed for quite other reasons—to unify parts of an emerging academic health center at Dartmouth, for example, or to maintain excellence in research and service at UCSF—find themselves, to everyone's surprise (including their own), soon immersed in and dedicated to curriculum reform. Finally, the propulsive effects of government- and foundation-supplied seed money, of the experimental approach to implementing change, and of a well-timed faculty retreat or workshop are demonstrated more than once in these chapters.

CHAPTER 4

Impetus

Left to themselves, institutions tend to persist in established practices. Combinations of outside forces and inside actors vested in change periodically disrupt equilibrium, however, prompting experiments and new practices perceived to be better adapted to evolving needs and thereby realigning the distribution of internal resources. The need to adapt—so as to survive, endure, or prosper, as the case may be—is the impetus for change. Sponsorship is related to impetus in the way that certain individuals inside institutions get the message and take the charge. Working from the top-down or from the bottom-up, depending on where they are placed, they announce the needs, set the goals, and, against more or less resistance, marshall the means. These individuals are the sponsors of change.

At Mercer, where a new school was created out of a local medical society, impetus came in the late 1960s from a U.S. congressman, a group of Macon family practitioners, and the local chamber of commerce's belief that central Georgia might well employ locally trained family physicians. The university eventually agreed to three-way sponsorship with the city and state, and, against outside counsel, a new medical school was in operation by the early 1980s.

- The whole thing got started in the late 1960s. At that time there were three forces in play. First, Congressman Carl Vinson wanted a medical school for mid-Georgia. He used the Health Professions Education Act that was passed in the late 1960s to build medical schools. Second, there was the local medical society in Macon, which wanted a school to train family-medicine practitioners. Third, there was the Macon Chamber of Commerce, which Vinson interested in the idea. Vinson got Nixon committed to our project, but then Watergate slowed the whole thing down. Finally, Vinson, the Medical Society, and the Chamber of Commerce got together and asked Mercer to be the academic home of the new mid-Georgia medical school. The university said, "No, we cannot afford it alone," and proposed a partnership between the medical center, the state, and the university. The medical school was eventually founded as just such a partnership. All the consultants at the time, from Vanderbilt, Southern Florida, and others, said, "Don't do it! You won't make it!" And it is certainly true that from the founding in the early 1980s through the mid-1980s it was very rough going.

Received record, the blueprint for change at Mercer came first from McMaster, then Michigan State recruits, the latter led by a strong dean who broadened the school's mission beyond family practice.

• The initial people here were from McMaster. The first crew trained and came from McMaster. These were people with a family-practice/primary-care orientation. Really the problem-based curriculum is a hybrid between McMaster, Michigan State, and Illinois. At one point the school could have become the largest family-practice program in the world. We have had six deans up to now. Bill Bristol . . . was the first to say that to be fully accredited we had to go broader than just family medicine. Bristol was the first strong academic dean. Until then the school was just a handful of guys in a few courses in basic science and clinical medicine. They were just a group of local people doing their politicking, and their politicking was family practice. The McMaster people came in before I arrived in 1979–1980. Before that it was all John Tripp. Bernard was dean for a while, a basic scientist with a PhD. Bristol came in around 1980–1981 when the building was about done. At Michigan State he had been the assistant head of the program in Kalamazoo. Bristol hired another guy from Michigan State, Paul Warner, who was assistant dean for curriculum. Until then, the McMaster people had control of the curriculum. Warner had run the Michigan State program in the upper peninsula. He was a medical education liberal. That is when the first curriculum was developed. It was a Michigan State and McMaster product.

At Hawaii, impetus came from latent opportunity, in the school's monopoly on in-state physician education, hence its room to maneuver, even across the Pacific basin. Sponsors appeared in a newly elected internal dean and his several long-standing colleagues in clinical medicine. The group possessed decades of experience in clinical instruction and island health care, strong awareness available to late innovators of what had been tried elsewhere, and a palpable sense of having long waited for the change moment to arrive at a very traditional medical school. The blueprint for across-the-board change, even an entirely new syllabus, came primarily from McMaster.

- It started with the new dean and a cadre of people who felt the same way about medical education. Gulbrandson was a professor of medicine here for 20 years. He became acting dean at first and then, after the search, was appointed dean. [I: Who were the catalysts?] Christian Gulbrandson, Alexander Anderson, who has been here for many years, and Max Botticelli, also here for many years. They are all in the department of medicine. They were the initial forces. There was a group that went to the AAMC [American Association of Medical Colleges] meetings in San Diego on problem-based learning run by McMaster in the spring of 1988. This included the dean and a number of others. Then the dean sent basic science chairs to New Mexico to look at their program. [This gave me] a better idea of what problem-based learning was, but I do not know if I was sold. There are some positive aspects, but I had some concerns too [about] the manner that students would learn the basic sciences in problem-based learning. I agree with the idea that in the old curriculum we did have information overload. I am a strong believer in self-learning and problem solving.

Hawaii, like Dartmouth 2–year within recent memory and curricularly very traditional, had known several within-bounds change efforts before the new dean took command in the late 1980s.

- There are [several] reasons why things got started. First, basic science teaching faculty number no more than 10 to 15 people here, total, and the same people had been doing it since the beginning. We had been successful by national board standards, but most of us saw stress issues arising with the students. I was chair of the curriculum committee beginning in 1980 or 1982. We saw that the stress level and exam mentality of students was very high and it reminded me of when I was a student. So we did an experiment. We decided not to have a collision of exams on the same day for the first 2 years, and this reduced the level of stress significantly. The problem was that there was a group of students who always got behind in this way. So in a way we ended up with acute episodic stress in contrast to chronic episodic stress. And whichever way we did it, there was always an information overload problem.

    Second, in these years, the curriculum committee began a review of the junior and senior years. We wanted a course at the end of the fourth year to tie up loose ends. I became the coordinator of a new fourth-year review course. This is the only thing, in fact, that has carried over from the preproblem-based learning days here. There were two goals for the course. To keep students' attention, we set up senior seminars, for example, a series on ethics that featured discussions with on-line people. There were 5 half-day meetings in the ethics series concerning ethics and obstetrics, pediatrics, medicine, surgery, and psychiatry. To give students ideas about such practical issues as health insurance, disability, investing, and generally to sensitize them to issues that they would be bombarded with after they graduated, I did a very controversial seminar. I invited the business school to do it with me but they did not believe that it could not be done in two half-day sessions. So I used several insurance companies instead and it has worked better. The companies must agree that they will not exploit the situation, but still there is a soft-sell aspect. We also cover more mundane things like surviving as a first-year resident, facing lack of sleep and constipation, [as well as] how to complete a death certificate, child and spouse abuse, that sort of thing. Students just loved these sessions. I also asked HMSA [Hawaii Medical Services Association], which is the Blue Cross/Blue Shield outfit here, to give students an overview of medical practice in Hawaii. . . . So we had these kinds of experiences before the change to problem-based learning. This was part of our review of the junior and senior years.

Third, everyone was upset that the students were not using the library much. This was also before the changeover. I surveyed the students and found out that nearly half did not use the library at all. The faculty was upset, but I said to them, "Yes, it is because they do not have to. With problem-based learning, they would have to use it a lot." I made the point that if they do not know how to use the library, they would not be as apt to learn later, and they will be less prone to continuing education. Taking all this into consideration, we could see that the way we were teaching meant that we were trying to make everyone into baby specialists. So I was happy to go to the AAMC meeting in San Diego in the spring of 1988 with all the sessions on problem-based learning. It was hosted by McMaster. The title of the conference was, "How to Implement Change in Medical Schools." The acting dean, Gulbrandson, brought four or five of us to the meeting with him, including the now chief of medicine, the chair of biochemistry, a senior professor in anatomy, the chair of pharmacology, and me. Problem-based learning intrigued me as an effective way to get students at issues to narrow information overload.

At New Mexico, a low-population state's single medical school founded on the traditional model in the mid-1960s, impetus also came from the room to maneuver. Unlike Hawaii, however, the school innovated early and thus invented more than it borrowed. The invention—a primary-care curriculum in operation by the late 1970s—grew out of experiments in clinical education modeled on New Mexico State University's nursing program. Nor was change at New Mexico sponsored top-down by a messianic dean as it was at Hawaii but bottom-up from the tinkering of a few faculty, one of whom was inspired by his own residency at Case Western Reserve.

- There were only two of us who wanted change at first . . . Arthur Kaufman and me. I came with a clinical research background. I had thought about education since medical school. I had not much enjoyed medical school in a small southern university. At Case Western, where I did postgraduate studies, I was treated very differently. At Case Western we formed a subcommittee on education and looked at resident education in pediatrics. I came here in 1970 and started a primary-care pediatrics clinical education experiment. It was different. We invited first-year medical students right into pediatrics clinics and more than half the class participated. Soon, I was on various curriculum committees and soon I was doing research in medical education. I sought to define competencies in student physicians. I did a lot of videotaping. I brought this material back to the curriculum committee. I kept raising questions about what we are doing to the students. Finally, they just said, "Shut up and write it all down!" So, I did. That got me into even more trouble, of course. The dean put me on a committee to look at the organizational development of the institution, as a junior faculty member. It was still a small institution then and a lot of us were still very young. Later I was on the search committee for the new dean and, when Len Napolitano came in, he asked me to be assistant dean. He asked me to take a look at our clinical science teaching, and I was thrilled to do it. I was interested and I was vocal. This was about 1973. In the first 2 years there was just headache after headache in the curriculum committee in these matters. I learned how difficult it is to work within the system. I learned, therefore, that it is easier to go outside to develop a pilot project. I also learned how not to treat the faculty. In those years the curriculum committee tried to force a package through the faculty, and of course it crashed. That taught me how to interact with faculty. It taught me that you do not push. It taught me that you inform everyone very well, all the time. Later, with the primary-care curriculum change, we used up a whole forest of trees! We xeroxed too much. We informed everyone to a fault. In those years, I learned, inform, inform, inform.

Kaufman got involved in 1974 after a period working with the Indian Health Service in South Dakota. He came back in 1974 to join the new family-medicine department. I knew Arthur from his time here, before 1971–1972. So, Arthur took over the undergraduate education program in family medicine and tried some new courses that developed students' experiences in clinical electives in the first and second year. He was very creative; he involved faculty in teaching patient care and in research and administration in community outreach programs, prison farms, for example. We found that being involved in clinical electives in the first 2 years enhanced students' desire to learn the basic sciences. In 1969 we started an affirmative-action program here and took in a number of students who did not have strong intellectual capabilities. We wrestled with these problems but let them continue, which was a mistake. At the time I was involved in a statewide program that the nurses had created to give a bachelor of science in nursing degree that counted their previous experience. New Mexico State University was certainly more innovative than we were then and had a career-ladder program for nurses. I wanted a similar program for physicians, so that those who were less able in medical school might become physicians' assistants on the model of the nursing program. I wanted to create a program that in the first 2 years would teach preliminary basic science and clinical studies to train physicians' assistants with practical, salable skills and in the second 2 years would teach advanced basic sciences and clinical studies to train MDs. [I: Did that bear fruit?] Well, that is the primary-care curriculum ultimately! It never became that [ladder] actually, but it did come to incorporate much else from the model. The AMA [American Medical Association] only let us do the 4–year MD program, so that we were never really in the business of training physicians' assistants. Arthur went to the AMA and they said that we could not bastardize medical education by making it physicians'-assistant training. So we backed off the physicians'-assistant program and ended up with a very different MD program than we had had before. The LCME [Liaison Committee on Medical Education] approved us at 20 students. At the time, Senator Kennedy was on the AMA for controlling medical education too much. This probably helped us get approved and explains, perhaps, why they moved on it so quickly.

Fostering the sponsors' belief in their effort at New Mexico was mounting federal, state, and foundation concern as early as the early 1970s over how skewed physician populations were becoming. Timely foundation support and the backing of their dean also helped.

- By the early 1970s, there was federal concern for the maldistribution of physicians. In 1969–1970, for example, New Mexico ranked 49th in the number of primary-care doctors compared to specialists, and, of course, geographically most physicians concentrated in the urban areas. We had some friends, state-level administrators, and Arthur and I took our original ideas to them. There were other people involved at the time, like the assistant dean before me, Bill Wiese, who was similarly inclined and went back to family medicine after his deanship and established the Navajo Area Health Education Center. He then became chair of the family, community, and emergency medicine department. So, we got some support from the state for these programs and it gave us courage to go to the dean. He suggested applying for a planning grant. We then visited several foundations. Arthur happened to go through Battle Creek, Michigan, on his way to New York City, and the Kellogg Foundation was excited about our ideas. It was 1976. We received a $48,000 grant to put some of our ideas into practice. Fortunately the chair of the department of medicine was on sabbatical, otherwise he would have shot it down. By the time he came back we were doing it!

    [The dean] has really been above it all. He lets us go do it. He is very good in the traditional mode. He does not entirely understand problem-based learning, but he has been supportive throughout. He never was a reform flagwaver, so the reform was initiated by Arthur and me. It is

not Len's style to jump on the bandwagon, but he did encourage us to get a planning grant [and] he would bring in
state money at the end of the fiscal year to augment Kellogg Foundation grant money into the next year.

Minnesota's efforts in the 1980s to integrate basic-science
and clinical instruction were sponsored, as at New Mexico, by a
few faculty members who drew support from the dean against
the strong turf mentality of departments. Impetus came from
their awareness of how fragmented the school's predoctoral curriculum tends to be, left to the departments' own devices.

• We have a very strong basic-science department tradition
  at Minnesota. Even so, we have made some progress from a
  strictly turf-oriented to a broadly coordinated point of view.
  This is due in large part to the dean, who has dissociated
  particular departments' budget allocations from the number of curriculum hours that they control. So while some
  departments have held on to the traditional turf point of
  view, others have wanted to integrate their activities. Traditionally, there has been a strong basic-science council
  here composed of all the department heads for first-year
  curriculum matters. The council is open to all basic-science
  faculty and some have recently come in saying, "We ought
  to do things differently. We ought not to have neuroanatomy and neurophysiology as separate courses. Instead, we
  should have neuroscience people." Some faculty do care
  about this way of doing things. Another example is in biochemistry. The old director says that biochemistry is finished and that we should be doing more cell biology in biochemistry. So the course director, Dennis Livingston, came
  and talked about it to the basic-science council and they
  told him, "Go for it!" He spent 2 years planning the
  changes. All this had the blessing of the educational policy
  committee, and in fact they would like to have taken the
  credit for these changes. The stimulus was really individual faculty members coming in and asking to put together
  something in a new combination. It also mattered that the
  basic sciences council saw that there could be savings of
  hours this way in combining and coordinating courses, es-

pecially savings in lab hours. Still, it was certain individuals, and not a council or committee, who pushed the courses forward. Until these people came forward, you were viewed as a traitor in your department if you proposed giving up even 1 hour of curriculum time. [I: How has the new cell biology course affected other basic-science areas?] It has shown them that the integrating process has begun.

Case Western Reserve, first and most original innovator in the previous reform cycle, does not now innovate much in teaching and learning. Impetus for change is muted at Case Western Reserve because the future, in which it is feared school standing will be diminished by relative slippage in research excellence, weighs more than the past, when educational discourse and experiment were worthy, well-funded activities.

- Fundamentally . . . there is no long-term goal for any effort to involve the whole faculty here in medical education reform. Effort is spent instead on a certain number of immediate objectives rather than on a process of innovation. The emphasis in Dr. Ham's era was instead on the process. It was really spectacular here in the 1950s and 1960s. There were three arms to it then. First, there was Ham himself, who insisted on openness and involved as many faculty as he could; second, Harlan Wood, professor of biochemistry, who dragged the basic science faculty along with the reform, insisting that talk had to cease and change occur; third, Jack Caughey, still here, who was dean of students and broke the mold for admission. It was Caughey who decided to admit the oddballs, including people with other professional degrees. He also valued performance other than on exams and was an extremely forceful personality. It was at this time that general faculty meetings were open not only to associate and full professors but also to assistant professors and others designated by the department chairs. Meetings then became very interesting and medical education became the domain of the general faculty. [I: Is it still?] No, it is not, but this is not anyone's fault. The attention of the academic world is now on survival. [I: Since when?] The decision that education was occupying too much of faculty time came in 1982 with the dean, Richard Behrman, who was a professor of pediatrics.

I believe that there are three elements in the business of medical education. First is what you aspire for your students, second is what you aspire for science, and third is what you aspire for the public. Certainly the astonishing feature of 1952 at Western Reserve University School of Medicine is how it addressed all three of these things. The debate in those years would flow from one to the other very freely. Now clearly, the unmet need is for the third element. We just do not pay attention any longer to the public. You could argue that the association that we have with Henry Ford Hospital in Detroit is such an effort. We also run a large HMO [health maintenance organization], for example, where we do seminars on patient care and so forth. But we do not do nearly enough. Our involvement in public medicine amounts to a gesture and is not founded on any principle. It is not magnanimous in any way. Since the 1950s, how we address the science element, although it is bitterly complained about, has held fairly steady.

As for our attention to students, I would say that it has become taken for granted because it is a custom here and needs to be revived. [I: How?] For the first time we are now requiring our second-year students to take the national boards. Before this was an option because you could take the FLEX [Federal Licensing Examination] exam at the end of the fourth year. On the most recent administration of the national boards, 22% of our students failed. Failure occurred in all the subject areas and in all parts of the class, even though some groups, such as Black students and some parts of the curriculum, including the cardiovascular and renal sections, were at higher risk. Whether the student came in with a scientific background or not, or was older or younger, or held another professional degree or not did not make any difference. Six weeks later, at the very next committee on medical education meeting, the chair and the dean and others met representatives from the next second-year class to explain the problem and propose a plan of action.

Now part of a big financially strapped academic health center, many at Case Western Reserve want more to boost research stature and clinic revenue now than to innovate again in education.

- The institution has become too conservative since the revolution of the 1950s. [I: Why is that?] Because of the success of that revolution, at least until the mid-1970s. Since then, while there have been many reform attempts, we have not done as much as we might have. It is possible that the school is now somewhat more research oriented. [I: When did this change take place?] It was in the previous deanship, in the mid-1980s. Then there was a rejuvenation of the basic sciences and a whole new set of basic science chairs were recruited. It was then that basic science began to have a more molecular outlook. Before, it was more conventional metabolic and systems physiology.
- The economics of the school is now said to be the dominant consideration. You must recall that the faculty [in the 1950s] was only 10 to 20% what it is now. If there are now 120 full-time faculty, there were then at most 10. [Dr.] Ham . . . knew how buttoned-up and conservative the internists were . . . knew their view that there are certain things that one just does not do. Ham broke all that apart and insisted that people say what was on their minds. It was also true that during the 1950s NIH was giving money away and we received large grants from the Commonwealth Fund. The researchers simply took the time then to have discussions. [I: When did things change, and how did they change?] When Dan Horrigan followed Fred Robbins as chair of the committee on medical education. He thought that the committee should retire into the background. When I became chair of the committee in 1976, I thought that the Ham model was the way to go and I attempted to revive it. But the real change took place when Richard Behrman became dean in 1982. I knew then that Behrman thought Metropolitan General was to be the only community hospital in our system and that we were not going to make it into a Boston City Hospital with a Thorndike Lab and so forth. In fact, Behrman said to me that he had never been to a

school with so intense a preoccupation with medical education as Case Western. He thought that it was all too much. This was the turning point. I chaired the committee on medical education from 1976 to 1982 when Behrman came in. [I: Was there anything that he felt Case Western Reserve was too little occupied with?] Yes, with science, and he was right. By the early 1980s it was clear that we were mistaken in believing that the Case Western Reserve golden age of science would go on and on.

Impetus is blunted at Dartmouth by the sharp divide between two parts of a still very traditional curriculum. After a bruising battle between basic and clinical scientists in the 1960s, Dartmouth added 2 years' clinical instruction to its formerly 2–year biomedical sciences program in the 1970s. Now, location as much as legacy separates basic and clinical sciences and curbs Minnesota-style integration, as the school recently put several miles' distance between its two respective teaching sites.

- The faculty has known for a long time that it could do a better job . . . teaching, but here, too, consistent with the idea that it is impossible here any longer to do something really distinguished, faculty feel constrained by a number of factors. First, there is the traditional structure of the medical curriculum, the 2–plus-2–year basic sciences and clinical education calendar. At Dartmouth, this division has been particularly profound because of the historical fact of a devastating fight here in the 1960s between basic scientists and clinicians [which] drove a particularly deep wedge. That division . . . has been exacerbated as well by another factor, by having the clinical program be in the Hitchcock Clinic, which is a corporate entity whose values are very different from the medical school. Keep in mind that our medical center is only a decade old. The Hitchcock Clinic was established long before as a private practice group in the Upper Valley, one which attracted practitioners largely for lifestyle reasons. A second constraint and major contributor to the division between basic-science and clinical education at Dartmouth lies in the fact that the three entities that have come together to form the medical center historically have been absolutely separate, have had separate boards of trustees and separate management structures. Much has been accomplished here in the last decade in creating the new medical center and representatives of these three different entities have worked to align themselves in a very short period of time. But at the same time resource issues have made the alignment very difficult. It is against this background that faculty both recognize the need to do a better job in teaching and perceive the constraints.

As divided as Dartmouth is, impetus to innovate may yet emerge in the 4–year school's desire to keep the company that it kept until recently as a 2–year biomedical sciences feeder school to the Ivies. Sponsorship may have come inadvertently, in a new outside dean recently recruited for more bread-and-butter purposes, and advertently, in the recently established "new directions" committee.

- Curriculum reform is a high priority for the new dean. [I: Was he recruited with that in mind?] No. Recruitment of a dean with the objective of curriculum reform was not intended. [I: Rather it was to lead the transition to the new medical center in Lebanon, New Hampshire?] Yes. But curriculum is one of the ways of doing this. [I: Who else gets involved in curriculum reform?] Myself. And Jack Wennberg, for example. He brings a particular view of the importance of some "missing basic sciences," such as evaluation strategies for outcomes and the role of patient values and utilities for making medical decisions. His view is that to restructure a traditional biomedical model of medical education, patient needs must be better understood by students, physicians, and the patients themselves. He might say that a medical education must be underpinned by basic biomedical knowledge, certainly, but he would also cite evidence that this knowledge alone has led us into profound kinds of uncertainty. He might say that the proliferation of medical theory has increased and not decreased the level of uncertainty in health care and that therefore we need to develop curricula in which students understand that one of their roles is to follow the course of therapies that they prescribe. He would question the notion that the delegated decision model is at all functional in medicine. If most decisions are made for quality-of-life reasons, then the only viewpoint that is really relevant is the patient's view of the value of outcomes.

- [I: In 5 years will such views of the necessary shift in medical education be embodied at Dartmouth to any significant degree?] I think that a middle-ground response will occur and that we will succeed in incorporating some of these elements. These will include making issues of the medical uncertainty part of the curriculum and the central importance of patient utilities in medical decision making. We will be more explicitly living in the territory between recruiting and retaining traditional basic-science faculty and fostering and supporting faculty who represent Flexner's "second set of facts." If we succeed, we will have developed a culture in which the value of these two perspectives, biomedical and behavioral, is recognized, in which each recognizes the other and does not dismiss it. In any case, reform will have three aspects here: the curriculum context within the new directions committee, linkage of the curriculum with society inasmuch as the Koop Institute unfolds, and the governance issue among and between the three previously separate entities that are now forming the new medical center. And if we do not get the governance issue right, then the rest is a waste of time.

At Harvard, impetus for innovation came from a tradition that the school may be at once original and excellent in anything that it tries. Harvard, like McMaster in its own way, competes not only with select peers but also with its own self-image, and in so doing, provides its own impetus to change. As prime sponsor of the now generalized New Pathway, the current dean devoted his efforts to redefining excellence in that pursuit—general professional medical education—which commands the least part of the school's attention. The local innovation effort that he thus energized coincided with and influenced the current cycle reform movement, which found expression in the 1984 *GPEP Report.*

- When I began the job in 1977, and before I had actually arrived here, I thought a lot about what a new dean could undertake that was value-added and might make a difference in arguably the best medical school in the world. My conclusion was to undertake a fundamental reexamination of the nature of medical education. You must realize that educating students to the MD degree is only a minor part of the total activity of our medical faculty. It occupies something like 5% or less of the total effort of this huge faculty, which is primarily involved in research. Research, in fact, takes up about 60% of this faculty's effort. About 30% is devoted to specialty-oriented patient care, and about 10% to education. Of that 10%, half goes to other than medical student education, for example, the education of residents, fellows, and physicians in the continuing-education program. So I thought a lot about what to do to make it happen. I was not interested in another "curriculum reform." I had been involved in that at Duke and Chicago in previous incarnations. Although in both cases we did address significant issues in medical education, in both it seemed to me that it did not really reach to the fundaments of the problem. So at Harvard we did two things. First, we initiated a series of annual workshops for faculty to talk about educational issues. Second, we launched an annual symposium on medical education which covered such topics as the role of computers and other information-managing technology in medical education, or the interfaces of the medical school with premedical experiences in the colleges and postdoctoral residency programs in teaching hospitals. Simultaneously we started a group of academic societies to be extracurricular communities of students and faculty in which I hoped there would be enough interaction so that there could develop a growing desire to have at the fundamental issues. For example, a clearer articulation of attitudes and skills as well as the frameworks of knowledge that all doctors, independent of their field and specialty, should share at the close of their course of education. I believe that, of these, attitudes are the most important, skills next, and then knowledge. The fundamental question is: How can these best be developed? [I: Your formulation was one of the precursors to the GPEP report?] Yes, I debated accepting the invitation to join the GPEP group. I wondered whether it would be a distraction or a help to the process here. I decided the latter and thus spent more than a little time with Steve Muller and that interesting group starting in 1980.

Innovation found impetus in a glaring contradiction at the University of California, San Francisco (UCSF). Grown accustomed by the mid-1980s to excellence in biomedical research and clinical service, the school was shocked at the same time to find itself failing in medical education. Quickened by crisis manifested in a student strike and a suicide, the new dean, thought to be only research oriented, came to sponsor a deep reformulation of teaching practice and admissions policy. Emboldened as at Harvard, many educators, formerly hidden in a school as discipline-department dominated as Minnesota, came forward.

- In 1983 . . . two things happened. First, there was a strike. Fifty-seven of 141 students refused to take the comprehensive medical exam at the end of the second year. It was a problem-solving exam, but the students only wrote essays on why the exam was unnecessary. That was a real shock. It forced a make-up exam. At a faculty meeting it was agreed that it was intolerable for the students to dictate to the faculty how to carry out the mission of the school. In the aftermath, I told the faculty, we must examine why this happened. Second, an excellent Black student committed suicide. He was in the second half of the second year at a high-pressure time. The reaction to this tragedy was overwhelming. Classes were canceled for a week. I had a committee formed to listen to the students over the next 6 months. What emerged was a realization of their intense dislike of the instruction given by basic scientists! And UCSF had and has one of the best basic-science faculties in the country! The basic-science faculty complained that stu-

dents were not interested or interesting. So they had younger faculty lecture to the medical students. Lectures were
attended by five to 10 students, while the rest just read
from the syllabus. Something had to give. And there were
many too many lectures. The complaints were bad teaching, inadequate coverage, and seven or eight lectures a day.
It became clear to me that we had to do something or there
would be a disaster. It hurt me particularly that we had a
superbly qualified faculty in the basic sciences, but that
the students were not receiving the educational benefit of
that faculty.

The McMaster MD program was founded problem-based in
the 1960s, at the very start of the current reform cycle. Like
Case Western Reserve in the 1950s, it was there at the start. By
the early 1980s, impetus for change came from the province's
medically disgruntled population and diminished economy. It
also arose from sharper resource competition with the school's
older, bigger competitor in Toronto. Internally, the program was
facing problems, known later at Mercer, of postdoctoral structures that remained naive or even hostile to its innovation in
predoctoral education. The 1983 "readjustment of chains" that
came in response was sponsored by administrators who read the
change underway in society.

- Let me remind you of the very different context at McMaster. In 1969 we were already doing what the *GPEP Report*
  was to recommend in 1984. Over time, we discovered that
  we were not able to change the postgraduate medical education program to be consistent with the MD program,
  thus that there are always limits to reform in the structural environment. For the MD program this has meant
  limits imposed by the postgraduate medical education program, but also, and more immediately, by the financial resource crunch of the early 1980s. Change is really a readjustment of the chains therefore. In 1983, this meant
  developing the "road-map" curriculum, which was a redefining in a more formal way of what it was that we wanted
  students to know. In the early 1980s we were recognizing
  that economic good times were not going to last forever. In

Canada we were seeing down the road the social changes that were coming as a result of the economic downturn. The Ontario health-insurance plan of the middle and late 1960s meant that doctors over the course of the 1970s were increasingly better rewarded. By the late 1970s the government was complaining about the enrichment of doctors. Ironically, these changes were favoring the McMaster sort of education, at the same time that our resources were being cut by the provincial government. There is also the context of the medical professional environment in Ontario. There are five medical schools in Ontario, and 45 miles from here there is the biggest medical school in North America. The University of Toronto Medical School admits 240 students a year in a 4–year program, and that perverts everything, including medical school politics, residency politics, and physician distribution politics. [I: Does this explain why McMaster seems to be looking over its shoulder quite often?] Yes, we have to. Let me give you an example. There is a Council of Ontario Faculties of Medicine. Its meetings include the deans of the medical schools and various satellite people. The group as a whole has faced a 10% cut in support for residency programs and now faces the same sort of cuts for other programs as well. When you are as big as the University of Toronto, however, there is an immense gravity that you exert on program funds, and so we must constantly be fending for ourselves at the provincial level.

At Sherbrooke, impetus for the mid-1980s changeover to problem-based learning and community medicine also came in part from provincial economic downturns, one severe enough to call the faculty's very existence into question, and at Sherbrooke, too, the change was sponsored top-down by top administrators and selected faculty members. Many, reportedly, recognized how sclerotic the curriculum had become.

- There were several reasons [why people wanted to change the educational program]. First, there was a clear perception here from a series of young faculty that the curriculum was not doing the job right. These faculty had catalogued a whole series of curriculum problems. The curriculum had become subject to a sort of chronic aging disease. It had become a "curriculum pathique." [I: Who were these young faculty?] They were people around me, but they had been talking together before I came here. There was a consensus building that poor teaching at Sherbrooke was creating poor students. The problem was identified as a system problem, not a people problem nor a teacher or student problem. [Second,] people knew that the social position of the Sherbrooke medical faculty had been lost. From 1970, when we graduated our first student, to 1980, it was a very innovative period, but then the innovation left with the people. By 1980–1981, there was a reversion to tradition here. Then in 1981, the university entered into a grave money crisis, and many positions were cut universitywide. This jeopardized the position of the faculty, which had been founded in the 1960s because of the need for more physicians. By 1980, it appeared to many in the province that there were too many medical schools, and that one of the four might be cut. [I: So you needed to redefine your niche.] Exactly. [Third,] Dean Pigeon. Pigeon was the dean under which the reversion had occurred. He went on sabbatical after serving as dean from 1979–1983. His daughter went through the medical school at just that time. Thus, the dean saw in his own family the medical education process change. In 1983 he was asked to come back as dean and in June 1984 he said that undergraduate medical education reform was the base of his mandate. [I: Was anything going on outside the school in these years that fostered the need for change?] Yes, there was definitely an evolution going on in medical educaxtion. People were trying new things. As early as 1976, I had founded the *Club de Pedagogie Medicale de Quebec* in order to bring the innovators together to share ideas and to consult. We have been meeting biannually ever since. By the time the *GPEP Report* came out in 1984, we used it to prioritize our needs. At Sherbrooke before and after I came in 1986, people were well-informed with these developments.

• Internally, everyone at the time wanted 1 more week of lectures to keep pace with knowledge in their own fields. In effect, we wanted to teach everything to everyone. We were beginning to need 7 years. Then too there were several previous attempts at renewal. In 1978 and 1982 there were committees established with charges to review and recommend. One of the recommendations was to add teaching time to the undergraduate curriculum. Then a third committee reversed the trend, and recommended instead lengthening the program to adopt a problem-based, student-centered, humanistic, community-oriented curriculum. [I: Any external circumstances?] Yes, every other year they were threatening to close the medical faculty at Sherbrooke. This gave us a very bad mood. It was a matter of survival. We knew that when you are the smallest medical faculty you have to be better than the others. Before the LCME touches a big medical school like McGill or the University of Montreal or Toronto or British Columbia, it must really be in default. For one of these schools, your faults have to be much bigger to be closed. [I: And being a smaller faculty?] You are much more easily closed. It is easier to be severe with a small school. This threat was the greatest around 1980.

- Dean Pigeon was the main force, and there were a few others. Leadership was a tremendous factor. Pigeon was the visionary, even though few people knew him as a teacher or clinician. I knew him in both roles, since he brought me here in 1969. He was a nephrologist at Verdun Hospital. I was interning there and he invited me to come to Sherbrooke as a resident. He is the reason why I am in general internal medicine. If the trend in Canada is to train physicians in general internal medicine, then Sherbrooke and Pigeon were very much part of this in the role modeling that they provided. We were early innovators in this. It was Pigeon's vision; it was his idea to treat the whole human being, not just the patient, he said then. And he said the same thing with respect to students.
- By 1980 . . . it was said that one medical school would be sacrificed, and that we were the youngest and smallest and therefore the most vulnerable. We were under a Damoclean sword. The dean said, "We have to do something, or we will not be around in 5 years." The *GPEP Report* came out at

about the same time, and right away we picked up these ideas. We saw many of the GPEP recommendations as a way out of the impasse. We jumped on board the new method for the sake of survival. It is a method, after all, that will produce adequate students for the province of Quebec.

CHAPTER **5**

Design

Innovative ideas well up from inside and cross over from outside institutions. They are often some cross-product of invention from within, a result of functional readjustments at various places in the institution, and diffusion from without. Those who think through how these ideas might be combined on-site become the designers of innovation.

Scope is related to design in that the configuration of change depends on who conceives it. Working top-down, a dean, or those with decanal blessing, may conceive change broadly, change that reaches across one or several rows, down a column, or even, more complicated, across the entire institution. Working bottom-up, even top-sanctioned, innovators conceive more circumscribed, within-bounds, change that is simpler and less fraught in the implementation. The location and sponsorship of those who conceive innovation, then, often determines its scope.

At Mercer the designers began blank slate in the late 1970s, and the ideas came by diffusion, first from McMaster, then from Michigan State. The sponsors' first charge, to conceive a school for training family practitioners, was soon exceeded by a strong out-of-state dean who broadened the scope beyond family practice. Curriculum was then redesigned top-down by Michigan State people who made sure that it did not depart so much from established practice as to risk favor with accreditors.

- [Bristol and Warner] wrote a syllabus which was huge and unwieldy. The head of the LCME [Liaison Committee on Medical Education], Jim Scofield, was opposed to problem-based learning and put them through a wringer. Andy

Hunt was dean at Michigan State and Warner was a student of his. It was Hunt who started the revolution in two tracks there. Scofield and Hunt were at each other's throats. Even though by 1980–1981 the experimental track at Michigan State was beyond question, since both tracks were working by then, Scofield was still fighting it. I left in the middle of that fight to come to Mercer and every battle I have gone through here I had gone through already at Michigan State! Warner and the Michigan State people who came to Macon decided not to resist the national boards. Warner said, "Do not fight the LCME. We have something good here. It is tested. It works. The experiment has been done at Illinois and Michigan State. Why fight the LCME? They say, Do the boards, so we will do the boards! The students who cannot pass the boards should not be turned out in any case, in all probability." When Bristol came, he was a superb internal dean. He hired most of the basic scientists and really got the school started. It was Bristol who put it altogether. He got the LCME in. He got the building done. He got the first class chosen. He got state money in line. He concentrated internally and angered some because he said "No" to virtually no one. So Bill Bristol got the school started. After 2 or 3 years, however, to the Georgia politicians, Bill was an outsider. Georgia is a place where you talk in generations, not in decades. Bill was a loving, caring, northern, blue-collar kind of guy. Soon we needed just the opposite and we were lucky to find Doug Skelton.

To defend against upstart Mercer's detractors, some of whom, as at Sherbrooke, wanted the school closed, an equally forceful in-state dean was broght in in the mid-1980s who, in turn, broadened the definition of primary-care training and put the school on firmer financial footing.

- The medical school at Emory [University] has a very traditional faculty and a lot of history. Likewise the medical college in Augusta was very well established. Many were trying to keep this place down. Some even wanted it closed. At Emory, Skelton was a traditional faculty member. He was just beginning to read about problem-based learning. Doug is a Mercer graduate who does not get much into the teaching part at the medical school. He is an excellent external dean. Even so he has gone around the country spreading the message of general professional medical education. Doug's agenda for the school has been based on the fact that two-thirds of the state's physicians are in Atlanta in the north, while 50% of the state's population is south of Atlanta. This is his point of view independent of problem-based learning. This is his political point of view, and this is why he supported the founding of the Mercer University School of Medicine when he was a university trustee. At the same time he was a faculty member at Emory. Doug has said very clearly that we will do what the state defines as primary care. That definition includes not only family medicine but also primary internal medicine, pediatrics, ob–gyn, general surgery, and general psychiatry. Skelton said, "These six are our mission, and I do not want to hear any complaints." To expand this way you need more political sensitivity than Bristol had. [I: So you had the right, people at the right times in both cases, Bristol and Skelton?] Yes, both of them. And that is about where we are right now. Predictably, we have just had a fuss with our students in this regard. Twenty percent of our recent class was applying for nonmission-compliant residencies. Doug blew his top. He wrote a memo, stating that we do not accept students who are not mission compliant. It is serious business with him. He has taken some heat about this. He is writing the residency directors to check on the integrity of students. He does not like our graduates applying for a primary-care residency and then doing radiology.

At Hawaii in the late 1980s, a new and dominant inside dean took charge of designing a broad-scope, McMaster-inspired changeover that was to span the entire 4–year program. Design effort conducted top-down benefits from a unified concept, but it also risks leaving out less-enthusiastic faculty, at Hawaii certain basic scientists who had already been innovating ground-up. These, at a small service-oriented medical school, would soon be needed to implement the change.

- The first thing we did was to designate . . . the MD planning committee [which then] became the MD program committee. I appointed everyone. People, high-powered people, the same people whom I organized when I was convincing people to make the change in the late 1980s. These were department chairs, respected educators, important clinicians, and MD students from each year. [I: Were the students voting members?] Yes, I let the students vote, because I made the decisions! In fact every committee at the medical school is advisory to the dean. I started out as chair of the committee and then I appointed a chair. [I: Strong dean tradition?] Yes, right from the beginning. [I: Why is that?] I will speculate. Politics and government in the state is highly centralized. Our governor is probably the most powerful in the United States. Keep in mind that Hawaii was a monarchy only 100 years ago. And until recently the "big five" plantations controlled everything. . . . That is how the various governors related to them, even Sanford Dole. So there has always been strong central government in Hawaii, meaning one department of health for the entire state, one department of education, one university, one medical school, one dean. The dean before me, Terry Rogers, served in the RAF. He ran this place like a battalion. He established this school by force of his personality. In our last site visit by the LCME, they dinged us on faculty governance—for not having any. This was the only thing they complained about. My view is that faculty governance is a help in the long term and a hindrance in the short term. I do not think that they will get organized while I am dean. I said to the faculty governance committee once, "Look, any well-run organization needs not only a mission but a value statement." They said, "What is a value statement?" The faculty here is a collectivity of individuals which is very little aggregated. The faculty committee is elected by each department. The way it turns out is that departments choose people because they have the smallest workload in the department!
- We invited Bill Shragge from McMaster to do a demonstration in the fall of 1988. It was a smashing success. We took a range of students and showed faculty that they did fine with problem-based learning. Shragge is incredibly gifted and has a sixth sense for things in tutorial, that is on the

stage. The dean had faculty sign what amounted to a document of intent. There were 50 or 60 people at the demonstration and 70 or 80% of them were basic scientists. The dean asked for a vote on whether it was a good thing to do or not, a written vote. Better than 95% said yes. Still, some felt that it was a bit coercive. The dean then had the chairs meet to draw up an implementation plan. We put together the plan and voted unanimously as department chairs to go ahead for the fall of 1989. And this was March 1989!

- I do not think that there was any strong feeling to change, as a general thing. How it came about is that the dean had a workshop on problem-based learning and invited Shragge from McMaster. He is such a charismatic person. He put on a nice demonstration. At the end he had people fill out a questionnaire that included the question, "Would you be willing to tutor in the first 2 years?" Forty people said yes. But it was not a vote to change the curriculum [though] the dean's feeling was that this was consent to change the curriculum. . . . [I: How many faculty attended the workshop?] Fifty to 60, mostly basic scientists. [I: Did you say that you would tutor?] Yes, I think that I did . . . but my interpretation is, Who was going to say that they were unwilling to tutor if you had that curriculum?

- A significant number felt that we were doing pretty well as it was. Their view was, "if it is not broken, don't fix it." This was especially so in pharmacology, since, of all the departments, they were always first or second on the national boards. We were right behind them, though. They did teach a marvelous course and it was very innovative, computer-assisted, and so forth. So a few key people in each department were skeptical [and some] thought that it was not a good idea to do it at all at first. I admit that it was a big faith issue. I could see that, to accomplish what we had set out in March for the following fall, we could not design all the cases ourselves. Thus McMaster sent us all their problems for the first five units lock, stock, and barrel.

New Mexico, where during the 1970s a few determined innovators worked up from below, illustrates both importance of support from above and the utility of creating an experimental track

to parallel, not replace, the traditional one. Choosing to design a
new column, as Harvard would, rather than innovate more mod-
estly as Minnesota or more ambitiously as Hawaii would, innovators at New Mexico developed a protected lab for untried ideas that
eventually yielded the school's primary-care curriculum.

- There were three of us ... Arthur Kaufman, myself, and
  Dayton Voorhees. He is no longer here, has a practice in
  town. [I: What did the group actually do, program design,
  course design, cost estimating, implementation planning,
  course approval, evaluation planning?] Any and all of the
  above. At first, we were the CPC, or curriculum for primary
  care group. Then, in 1977–1978, for 3 or 4 months we were
  the RPC, or rural primary care group, but in that guise we
  were shot down when we went out around the state to get
  support. We found out that nobody wants to be called rural.
  Then we were the PCC, or primary care curriculum group.
  At first, our friends thought these efforts were okay and
  the rest thought, well, if you just ignore them, they will go
  away. So, a small group came to work with us and others
  were not bothered much. The administration was supportive. The dean had the view that, well, this will not hurt. He
  said, "Let's take it to the chairs. Let's get a planning
  grant." He was supportive and that support did not go
  away. In the fall of 1977 after an 18–month planning grant,
  we applied for implementation money and received
  $700,000 for 3 years. We did the budget then and worked
  the faculty, trying to get as much support as we could. We
  developed a blueprint for turning out primary-care physicians and were effective enough so that, at the largest faculty meeting ever held at this school, in September 1977,
  our proposal passed without one dissenting vote. We did a
  good job in the care and feeding of faculty, and the next
  September we turned to the students. [I: Any off-campus
  advice and information?] We brought in a very talented
  guy who had put together the planning for the Alaska
  pipeline, as a matter of fact, a systems theorist named
  David Halcomb [with whom] we designed all the charts and
  plans that really impressed the grantors like Kellogg. [I:
  Main points of agreement and disagreement within the

group?] I do not even remember. It all got worked out, although disagreement still exists. . . . As for agreement, there has always been consensus on the basic philosophy of educating medical students. We recommended a pilot program with 20 students that we then got the LCME to approve.

Only in recent foundation-funded redesign efforts to integrate the best of both tracks has real discord, dodged to date by the parallel track arrangement, arisen.

- If politics is the art of compromise, then we have not been good at compromising recently, in the sense that we have given on way too much. We so much need this thing to work, to integrate the PCC and traditional tracks under the Robert Wood Johnson grant, that we have promised everything. This is potentially our downfall, I would say. Still, the opponents are few, numbering less than a dozen. It is a small group of faculty that is providing the major engine for this. [I: In hindsight, would you do anything differently?] Personally, hell yes, but generally no. My style is far more structured compared to Kaufman's, which is more open-ended. I would have introduced more structure into the design process. Faculty are not exactly asking how we are going to get more structure into the program. Many fear central control and find it easier when nobody works for anybody. They prefer consensus management, which in my view works only selectively, the common idea that everybody wants their own little fiefdom in the university. Less structure can work when there are only 20 of 73 students in the primary-care curriculum. Now, when the two programs are to be integrated and all these things have to work together, it is another matter. We still do not know the answer to the problem of loss of control and power for those who have resisted central control until now. There is no question, for example, that I have accrued significant power in the process of implementing the primary-care curriculum and that I am seeking now to integrate it with the Robert Wood Johnson Foundation grant. I have . . . more staff than the dean has, in this. So a lot of people are jeal-

ous of me and see me as a threat. The institution can no
longer operate in small fiefs with the global change that is
taking place.

At Minnesota since the mid-1980s, designers of alternatives to turf-segregated basic-sciences instruction have likewise
worked hard from below and found support from above. In contrast to New Mexico, however, the Minnesotans have been bound
by an unwritten rule, which limits the scope of innovation, according to which curriculum change must be brokered at the pe-
riphery, not promoted or protected from the center. Innovation
for this reason is both tenuous and of more limited scope at Minnesota.

- I am sort of a broker in banking hours among the basic-science departments. I am the coordinator of the first-year basic sciences. I meet with course directors, and my meetings
  are not always smooth. [I: Where are the rough spots?] Getting faculty comfortable with each other, for example, in
  the neurosciences. Questions arise about who lectures, an
  anatomist or a physiologist or someone else, on the subject
  of pain, for example. It is hard to find course directors to
  really hold their people together. While I have been coordinating the basic sciences, we have gone through several
  course directors in the process. This year we have chosen to
  do segments of pharmacology throughout the first year, but
  students find this very difficult, and so pharmacology may
  well become part of the neurosciences or of physiology,
  taught, for example, along with renal or cardiovascular.
  The new head of pharmacology likewise has the point of
  view that it is better to integrate and coordinate than to
  ask simply, how many hours do we get? In fact, many department heads are not going after hours any more, in part
  because now we have to teach not only medical students
  but also dental and nursing students. In these circumstances, you have to integrate and change. But it is also
  true that if someone like the dean or the legislature were
  to say that the existence of your department depends on
  the number of curriculum hours, then boom, the coordina-

tion game is over, and you have to meet the payroll. [I: Then this is all very tenuous?] Yes, it is.

Those who might have conceived educational innovation at Case Western Reserve were hampered by the school's mounting research- and clinic-revenue preoccupation throughout the 1980s. By the time new leadership had introduced the changes necessary to fill beds and balance books, few felt compelled to discuss, let alone design, innovation in either the old Dr. Ham or the new GPEP lexicon. The 1990s preoccupation with regaining biomedical science research stature serves similarly to restrain those who might currently rethink education method and content.

- Behrman, the new dean, formerly a professor of pediatrics, introduced a very strong money orientation. This wiped out a significant number of distinguished faculty members who found it very unpleasant and just left. At the same time the department of medicine found a new chair . . . a really splendid person appointed because he had a plan for the department to become solvent. Under Otel Mahmoud it now ranks in the top 20 in the country for NIH [National Institutes of Health] grants. With his efforts, funding has increased dramatically, and the department has continued to attract good residents. On the other hand, he has little concept of how to stimulate the education program. So the sea change, I would say, began with Little's appreciation that the university hospitals were desperate. The good news is that beds are now full at Lakeside, Babies' and Children's, and McDonald's Hospitals. [I: Any bad news?] I do not want to overstate things, but I think that the cost was diminished attention to the intellectual or nontechnical parts of medical education as well as almost complete lack of consideration of where the profession is going, where care of the public is going. I am increasingly concerned about this. Only very recently at Lakeside Hospital, for example, in our conferences on morbidity and mortality, have we succeeded in putting into discussion such public and medical ethics issues as the problems of drug addiction or of spending in the last year of people's lives. Only at

Metropolitan is a study currently under way of how the
sickest people get care. At the university hospitals, such as
Lakeside, this gets no attention. So here we are at a time
when a new national system of medical care will be devised
in the next 4 years, yet nobody in the medical school or in
the teaching hospital is discussing how to change accordingly. Even at Huff Norwood Hospital, all I hear is that we
are not going to be guinea pigs in community-care medicine. [I: Then there are many barriers?] Yes, the problem is
to get a forum inside the medical school to discuss new
health care delivery systems. We are hardly tapping this
and so the primary model of ambulatory care medicine is
still the outpatient clinic, which is a very clumsy way of delivering care.

For all that stands against it at Dartmouth, and as individually sponsored as it may have been, there is considerable scope
to recent change in clerkship instruction brought by the efforts
of a clever junior administrator intent on putting more students
in outpatient settings. As at Minnesota, the change at Dartmouth was more brokered than designed outright.

- I was given a job in 1986 as assistant dean of clinical education. The academic dean then, said, "Fix our clerkship
  schedule." That schedule was on the Dartmouth College
  calendar, which meant that everything was screwed up. I
  took all the clinical people on the curriculum committee
  and said, "Look you all, we should get on to the same
  schedule as other schools, for example, Harvard, so that it
  is easier for our students to go away for electives." So we
  reviewed each clerkship and those that requested more
  time got it, but only in exchange, I said, for putting 25% of
  it in an outpatient setting. I was tricky! All clerkships except for neurology and psychiatry wanted more time in the
  third year. Psychiatry was at 8 weeks and knew that they
  could not get more. Medicine and surgery were each at 10
  and wanted 12. I said, "Explain to me why you want the increase and how you will meet the requirement for an outpatient setting." It took 3 years but in the end the package
  covered the whole of the third and fourth years. And there

were students on the committee. I gave the students the power to negotiate how many weeks obstetrics, pediatrics, psychiatry, primary care, and all would get. The students negotiated it all. Medicine and surgery, for example, got 12 weeks. The students presented it to the curriculum committee. At the time, medicine went through a leadership change, which is why the process took so long. But the new chair, Sox, said okay. There was only one dissent on the curriculum committee and this is because psychiatry was cut from 8 to 7 weeks. I wrote a paper on the whole process for the "Power and Leadership" course at the Harvard Graduate School of Education. I asked why it happened at all and suggested that I was a woman acting in a zone of indifference working with male clerkship directors whose attitude was, "Just do your job and don't bother me." So with this indifference we made a humdinger of a change. The clerkship directors decided not to bring it to the faculty for passage. So I just presented it at a faculty meeting and everyone clapped! The following year we had meetings every month or 6 weeks for each director to present results. By the end of the year, psychology and neurology wanted to do it too. It was the bandwagon effect.

It is arguable that such individually invented, personally brokered efforts are more effective at schools like Dartmouth and Minnesota, which have so little center, than the sort of schoolwide outside-informed design effort now under way at Dartmouth.

- When I first started thinking about creating the new directions committee, that was in November 1991, 15 months after I got here, I called [Harvard Dean] Tosteson and asked him, "How do you do it?" He said, "Identify a small group of highly respected people who can think about the total experience and not just a piece of it." That is how I created the new directions committee. I picked Bill Culp, from the dean's office, who is highly respected for the way his head works, John Wennberg, who is a national leader in health care reform and outcomes research in the doctor–patient relationship, Martha Reagan-Smith, who has watched the education process more critically than anyone, Ken Burchard, a surgeon at the Hitchcock Clinic, who is also chair of the department and served on the American College of Surgery's task force on graduate medical education, and Elmer Pfefferkorn, acknowledged as one of our best teachers and highly regarded by everyone.

At Harvard the design effort was headed by the ranking administrator who, by position, could innovate top-down, first down a column by spurring conception of a new experimental society, later across-the-board by having its positive parts generalized across the entire predoctoral medical curriculum. The method that worked earlier at New Mexico, to experiment down a new column, worked at Harvard as well because, administration-sponsored, it soon engaged the efforts of many educators on the faculty.

- Dean Tosteson did it here and deserves the credit. He was awfully skillful getting the reform through. He brought it in as an experiment, and how can a medical faculty not accept an experiment? So there were 25 New Pathway students at the end of year 1 and 40 at the end of year 2.
- I started as Dean at Harvard in 1977 and by 1982 I grew impatient because the academic societies had relaxed into a happy but definitely extracurricular posture. So for the faculty workshop in the spring of 1982, I wrote a protocol and presented it. I said that we needed to do something more proactive. This resulted in a steering committee of senior faculty whose involvement and acceptance was essential to getting the thing off the ground. [I: What thing?] To form a society with responsibility and authority to educate its own students in a different way. This was the Oliver Wendell Holmes Society. So we did that, and the process involved this steering committee, which resulted, by the end of 1982, in an exercise in which subcommittees developed statements of the attitudes, skills, and knowledge that it seemed to us all doctors should share. Then, in the spring of 1983, the faculty council approved the recommendation of the steering committee that we prepare a plan to admit 25 students into the Holmes Society for the fall of 1985. We

engaged Dr. Gordon Moore as director of the New Pathway and then Dan Goodenough to be master of the society. In the spring of 1984 the curriculum was passed. By that spring, therefore, we could accept students in good faith into the New Pathway, because we then knew and so they knew what they were getting into. We accepted 25 students for 1985 and 30 for 1986.

In 1987, it became evident that there was more and more tension in the community between the ins and the outs. There was a tumultuous meeting of students in the spring of 1986, during which one student came to me and said, "What do you think my grandmother will think when she reads about the New Pathway, and I am not in it!" This is when we decided to accept all students for the New Pathway by providing three additional societies with curricula that were not identical to Holmes but strongly influenced by it. This resulted in a situation in which we retrogressed organizationally. What I mean is that, in a way, it made the societies extracurricular again, moving from a separate track with its own content into general use. Thus, in addition to the Holmes Society, we had Castle, Peabody, and Cannon. Of these, Castle was the new society. Peabody and Cannon had been in existence since 1978. Actually, there is a fifth group functioning as a society. From 1971, we have had the Harvard/MIT Division of Health Sciences and Technology. This has been an effort to bring into medicine more students with physical sciences and engineering backgrounds. Irving London, the first director of the program, generalized the Harvard/MIT program's approach to recruiting students who want to undertake any kind of biomedical research, like biochemistry, not limited to the physical or mathematical or engineering sciences. The Harvard/MIT Division's program leading to the MD degree has its own faculty, recruited from Harvard and from MIT. It has its own curriculum committee and administrative apparatus, and therefore many of the characteristics of the structure that I have wanted in the societies. The one difference, of course, is in programmatic focus, since the Harvard/MIT program is more limited in focus than is appropriate for the school of medicine as a whole. In 1992, we went back to the drawing board and by now have recruited a new team of masters charged with the responsibility to deliver the curriculum to the students in their societies. We have always resisted having the four societies differentiate by subspecialties in medicine. We want students in every society who can go into any field of medicine that they choose.

UCSF, like Harvard, benefited from the position and agility of its top administration, even though the scope of its innovation was not as broad. Eschewing a formal review of curriculum, a new "research dean" surprised many by deftly delegating a series of specific but highly consequential educational innovations starting in the mid-1980s.

• I did not want a formal curriculum review. I had been at Harvard when part of pathophysiology was introduced, and at the University of Chicago, and my feeling was that formal curriculum reviews produce a lot more heat than light and burn up a huge amount of committee work with little outcome. Therefore I started slowly, with a retreat in 1985. I assigned the two faculty members who were farthest apart on issues to one room. In this way I introduced chairs who had never met before. It had a very salutatory effect. I also soon realized that I needed professional help. I knew that this would be difficult since education is thought to be a faculty responsibility and faculty want to keep it away from the administration. Looking for help, I met Barbara Gastel at MIT. She has an MD from Hopkins, a BA from Yale, and an MS from Johns Hopkins in public health. She is the author of the book *How to Teach Science to the Public.* She was on leave as assistant professor at Peking University. I asked her to come in as assistant professor of teaching and teaching evaluation. It turned out to be a whopping success. From 1984 to 1989, she gave courses to faculty on how to teach, how to lecture. She gave four courses a year with 50 or 60 faculty at a time. She would take one basic-science course at a time and write a critique. Some of her critiques were scathing. . . .
    But I also looked at the way education issues were be-

ing handled by several committees and saw that each was working separately and often ineffectively. The committees were making decisions and passing pronouncements, but nothing was happening because the power for implementation lay with the department chairs. So I created an education policy and curriculum affairs committee and put all eight basic science chairs on it. It took some prodding. I had them form subcommittees on the clerkship and on basic sciences and so forth. In fact, the committee took on the job of setting up a new curriculum and monitoring it. I just did it and nobody asked any questions. There are still about four or five chairs on this key committee.

As nowhere else but Mercer, recasting admissions policy, though in quite a different manner, figured prominently into the change at UCSF.

- I also asked Holly Smith, who had just stepped down from being chair of medicine from 1964 to 1986, to be associate dean of admissions, [and] with Holly things changed very quickly. The class changed within a short period of time. It became younger, more science oriented, more achievement oriented. It was because of Holly that the 1989 accreditors said, "We have never seen a school where students are so happy." This was only 6 years after the strike! I do not want to give the impression that this process was all that planned. It was not. But we got much better when we had a better idea of what students needed.

UCSF illustrates how much can be accomplished piecemeal yet schoolwide when a skilled top-down player conceives the change. Like Minnesota, it also shows how difficult it is, due to differences in power base and reward structure, to reconcile turf-based department organization and schoolwide education innovation.

- First, Rudi brought in Barbara Gastel. She was a very good observer. She would sit in on basic-science classes and take notes. She did student opinion polls. She produced damning things about the basic sciences here. Second, Rudi restructured the curriculum committee. Third, Rudi focused on basic-science instruction and engaged some very dedicated people in the basic sciences, including Sexton Sutherland in anatomy, Diane Colby in biochemistry, and, in neurobiology, Warren Levinson, who switched from research to a teaching career. Rudi gave it full recognition and support. Levinson and I designed problem-based learning tutorials for a pilot of five and then 10 or 12 students. I went to the curriculum committee in 1986–1987 and they said, "Go ahead, no problem, but do not expect any money." After the pilot, the students said, "Great for the first year, now what about the second year?" Gastel started student teaching awards to bring teaching up to par and to praise people who did it well. There were meetings held and committees formed in this regard. For example, human genetics was getting dismal reviews each year. They got a visit from the dean, and the subcommittee of the curriculum committee was formed to review them. The committee does give great recommendations like more time, space, teachers, but we do not have real clout over the departments. None of this praising or implicit hand-slapping does any good if the department chairs do not help out. The next step, therefore, which we must take, is more vertical integration down through departments. But we have not done much beyond what I have just said. The department chairs are not radical reformers, but some people, like Colby in biochemistry, have had a big effect on their departments.

Curriculum redesign at McMaster in the early 1980s was conducted top-down by a combination of MD program administrators and faculty. What they conceived programwide was a more standardized curriculum than had obtained in the 1970s, one better suited to the 1980s' more practical ethos and larger student body, consisting of a new matrix of horizontal units and vertical perspectives and a new set of more community-based problems.

- Faculty were not particularly aware of us. There was no great beating of the drum among faculty. It was pretty much business as usual in the early 1980s. Indeed, there was a slow swing of the pendulum away from the left point of view. The clinicians became a little more conservative and began wanting more basic-science content. And everyone began evolving away from the idea of openness and direct feedback that characterized the 1970s. With Reagan's election in 1980 the handwriting was on the wall. The fiction at McMaster has always been that we want students to learn how, not what. But this of course is insane. You can easily go off the deep end this way and end up knowing more about the moon and the stars than how to help someone with hemorrhoids. Therefore we developed three perspectives that were to be infused throughout the units. Units and perspectives fit together in a matrix. The perspectives were first, population; second, behavioral; third, biological. We also tried to introduce uniformity and so in unit 2, for example, we had the head honcho get together with the subunit planners and coordinate what they were teaching. We also formalized the curriculum, made formal what previously had been informal in the student-based problem-centered learning approach. In these years, in the early 1980s with 100 students, you just could not do the things you did earlier with 20 or 40 students. This was the background to our efforts to make the curriculum more uniform and more formal. We are still almost apologetic about the ways we are changing as a result of experience. A good example is the student progress test that we have recently instituted. We think that our students will benefit from an assessment of how well they will perform on conventional tests. We think that they need a compass to know how they are doing [and] in this case I agree. . . . The purists, on the other hand, say that the progress test is out of step with the McMaster way. [I: They ignore that to stay the same, you must change?] Yes, the purist thing in problem-based learning is still very much here. At Harvard and New Mexico, the curriculum experiment is limited to tracks that go in tandem with traditional teaching. I think that the courageous thing is to change everything from the start. In my view, McMaster has not backed away from innovation.

There were specific products, more than actual recommendations. Foremost, these included written problems in health care and the establishment of community-based experiences for students. . . . [I: And the reactions?] There was no screaming, although there were a few dissatisfied people. We said, "Well, you modify it, then." The critics were also free to adapt the problems as they wished. It was always a matter of the traditional and older faculty who always had strong views about how it was done "when I was a resident in 1953." Vic Neufeld took the problems to the MD committee for revision. Subsequently they were presented to the health-sciences faculty education committee and then possibly to the senate. They were eventually approved and ratified by the faculty executive committee.

Underlying the formalization of curriculum change was growing interest at McMaster, spurred by 1980s provincial recession and the school's sense of unrealized mission, in how the "burden of illness" might be distributed across its population. Proponents, aided by tacit support from the dean and by the MD program's placement in a comprehensive health-sciences faculty, broadened curriculum scope to incorporate more clinical epidemiology. Their activity, as at Harvard, influenced the overarching design process that culminated in the *GPEP Report*.

- The whole basis of this revision grew out of the community-health-status review that was made by Vic Neufeld and other faculty, including Fran Scott at the department of public health. Neufeld's review was called "The Priorities, Problems, and Conditions Survey," or something like that. It was with this information that the curriculum revision was propelled and shaped. It was the architecture of the new curriculum. We loved the term "burden of illness." It means the impact on the community more broadly than just on the individual sufferer of a particular disease or condition. Thus the "burden of illness" would include consideration of a family's days of work lost, various economic spin-offs, and family dynamics cost in nonmonetary terms.
- Neufeld initiated the curricular review in the early 1980s. He was very interested in the health of the public, and this was before the Pew Charitable Trusts project. He was very

interested in the question, "What is the burden of illness in the city of Hamilton and in southwest Ontario?" and for that matter beyond. He asked, "Does our curriculum really incorporate clinical epidemiological data into medical education, for example, data concerning differential morbidity and mortality?" He decided that we had not done nearly enough. Neufeld was a leader in this, but not a boat-rocker. Concurrently, the central administration was in a maintenance mode, and this helped . . . allowing Neufeld and others to run with the ball. Neufeld's view was, "Do not ask permission, just do it and ask for forgiveness later." . . . There was also the historic role of the MD program here which attracted and continues to attract these sorts of people [and] the fact that we are a faculty of health sciences and thus have some collaboration between the various disciplines and professions, which is more fostering of health education. [I: Was the early 1980s a second wave of the McMaster movement?] No. The first was the wave, and this was just a ripple. This was almost as simple as a change in literature and in focus. It was really only the incorporating of macro-data into the curriculum. The principles and the approach of the program have long since been laid down. [I: And yet this little ripple had a big effect on the *GPEP Report.*] Yes. Vic Neufeld was the connection. We did sell ourselves well in the early days. In general, there was a growing acceptance here of epidemiological research, acceptance in the scientific medical community, acceptance of a focus on public issues, and the beginnings of MDs' acceptance of the kind of statistical research that speaks in terms of confidence intervals, *t*-values, and sample size. And beyond McMaster too, there was an advancement of the public health point of view at other schools. I would say that a global shift begins to occur in the early 1980s among some medical schools with respect to this focus on public issues.

At Sherbrooke, as at Hawaii, broad-scope departure from standard practice was conceived top-down using a blueprint from a host of earlier innovators in the present reform cycle. If most faculty began unconvinced or just unaware, many were

quickly and artfully co-opted into a deliberate, fast-paced design
process by a small group of forceful innovators who had the
threat of closure and the new *GPEP Report* working for them.

- Most faculty were either reluctant or unaware. The number of convinced faculty was very small at first. [But] let
  me step back . . . In September 1985, Dean Pigeon sent me
  to Egypt to a meeting of the Network of Community Oriented Educational Institutions for Health Sciences at the
  Institute for Health Science. It was part of my recruitment.
  On my side, I was asking, Who at Sherbrooke is ready to
  change? I did not want just a small group. I wanted a serious, unambiguous dean to lead this change and, in fact,
  Dean Pigeon considered it his mandate. He was really
  there for us. That was the beauty of it. I would say that in
  the mid-1980s the administration was more progressive
  than the faculty with respect to undergraduate medical education reform. Then, when I decided to come, I began by
  developing a nucleus of five people. This was in [late] 1985.
  The people included Dean Pigeon, Bertrand Dumais, Robert Eglesias, Danielle Bourgaux, and myself, an informal
  group around the dean. Next, we organized a bigger group
  to organize the framework of our change. We decided on 24
  people, 18 from different departments, 4 students, and 2 resource persons. We called it the "framework committee,"
  and we went through a 5–step sequence of planning, the
  first of which was to identify the characteristics we desired
  of our graduates. We gathered information on nine innovative institutions, including the medical faculties at the
  Maastricht, New Mexico, McMaster, Michigan State, and
  others. We divided the committee into groups and each
  group presented and defended the curriculum of one of the
  schools. Next we went from nine pairs of people to six tri-
  ads and we asked each group of three people to go home
  and to each develop from all these resources the new
  Sherbrooke curriculum. The conclusions that we drew from
  this exercise are almost the same as the curriculum that
  we now have. We agreed on the need to do something innovative and exciting . . . something to push out in front of
  medical education reform schools. We disagreed first on the

community orientation of the new program. It was very difficult, and I think that the conceptualization was not very clear, especially with respect to the implementation of a community orientation. We also disagreed on the subject of medical humanism, and there was a lot of ridicule inside the group concerning what some saw as an effort to create the barefoot doctor on the Chinese model for Sherbrooke graduates in Quebec. There were also some who thought there was not enough scientific content in the program as it was being designed. We had real debate in all these areas. There was also concern for the numbers of teachers and tutors required and for the numbers of rooms that the new program would need, that sort of thing.

- We started faculty development activities and raised the level of discussion about medical education in the years 1984–1986. Jean Jacques Gilbert from the World Health Organization came to do workshops for us. [But t]he landmark was hiring Jacques Des Marchais in 1986. Before, there was faculty development and some general reflection. After, there was still this but there was also more direction and focus . . . more active organization. We organized a canvas group and then invited 20-odd people to form a framework committee and assigned them in groups to study nine curricula . . . Maastricht, McMaster, New Mexico, Beer Shiva, Laval in Quebec, Michigan State, Southern Illinois, and a few others. Eventually we came up with a program based on this process that identified four characteristics around which we wanted to organize a new curriculum at Sherbrooke. We said that we wanted a curriculum centered on the patient, therefore a curriculum that was humanistic and community oriented. We also said that we wanted a curriculum centered on the student, therefore problem based and self-directed. The four characteristics were thus humanistic, community, problem-based, and self-directed learning. In truth, I was the one who made this synthesis and it was a very important summary of our process. Then in June 1986 the decision was made concerning whether to base the curriculum on organ system units or problems units. Some suggested 50 main problems, independent of organ systems. But the systems perspective prevailed. If we had not maintained an organ-systems perspective, the resistance to the change would have been huge. The canvas committee, which was made up of the core people, five or six in all, blasted through these major decisions and was then disbanded in June 1986. Then a smaller group, no more than two or three, took over to implement the program.

- For the faculty at large, the view was, "Why do we have to change at all?" Faculty saw that our students were succeeding quite well at the national level and wondered why there was any need to change. We answered that the changes we had in mind not only increased our chances for survival but also were in accord with the *GPEP Report* recommendations which were being promulgated in those years. GPEP really confirmed our track as we were envisioning it. [I: Were there any differences among faculty with respect to how they viewed the change?] There were. The basic scientists were against it from the start. Among the clinicians there was less opposition. I must say, though, that the visionaries, the several people who at first proposed the changes in the direction of problem-based and student-centered learning as well as the humanistic and community orientations, were very skillful. They had a lot of people like me against them. So what they did is put these people on the committee that explored the changes that they had in mind. They asked, "What would you do if you had to design a new curriculum along these lines?" It was what we called the "canvas of the curriculum," and in the process we established the scaffold, or the framework, of the new program.

- One thing that is sure. I am a family physician and an emergency-room physician. My attitude is, just do it! Des Marchais is an orthopedic surgeon, and so his attitude is likewise, just do it! Dumais is a cardiologist, and cardiologists have the same attitude as well. All three of us have a jump-in style. And we were the people who designed and implemented the program. The dean was always a source of major support. Dean Pigeon had been highly innovative for the 1970s and early 1980s. He knew that the key to survival was innovation when you are the smallest and youngest medical school in the province . . . knew, therefore, that we had to be different, that we had to be innovative, that we had to be ahead of the others in order to survive.

Having handpicked design committee members and steered their work toward adapting an outside blueprint to Sherbrooke requirements, the original group next sent itself and committee members out to sell their proposals to the departments and to secure broader faculty approval. With that approval, which came in stages, the group then pulled back in to prepare for implementation.

- At first it was very much an internal process. Only at the end of the process did we submit "le programme des études." I wrote it over Christmas 1986. In medicine, we are not used to working with people up and down the line. In fact, we did not even really feel accountable to the campus. I was very confident about the process. We had a sympathetic dean; I myself had been in this business since 1972; I was in tune with the trends; the world was evolving; and I knew that it was not just me. Dean Pigeon invited Vic Neufeld from McMaster to come to Sherbrooke. Neufeld had chaired one of the GPEP committees. Also Ron Richards, who had been my adviser at Michigan State University, had been working at the Kellogg Foundation before going to the Center for Educational Development at the University of Chicago, came for a visit. We also consulted Gilbert, who was the Director of Training Personnel at the World Health Organization in Geneva. [Then, consulting] the departments, our strategy was to listen but not to go into philosophical debate. We sought to communicate confidence in our strategy, a feeling that it would work. For myself, however, being as I am, it was very difficult for me to avoid argument. For me, this strategy of confidence was very conscious and was planned in advance. For Bertrand Dumais, there was not so much of a conscious strategy. The two of us, who were the principal leaders at this point, were very complimentary to each other therefore. In presenting the new program to the departments, we were very collaborative. After consulting the departments, we did not come back to the original group. The framework committee was an adjunct committee of 24 members that disbanded at this point. After that, the process was all in my office. It was pretty much Bertrand Dumais and Jacques Des Marchais. We began to plan the curriculum. We invited three or four persons from each unit in sequence. We gave them the mandate to develop that unit of the new curriculum. We gave them the mandate for the 12 points that that unit must cover.

- In the beginning, there was not a text, but rather a table of recommendations in the schematic form that I have already mentioned. One dimension was patient centered, in which we described a humanistic and a community orientation, and the other dimension was student centered, in which we described a problem-based and a self-directed learning format. Later, in 1986 and 1987, every document that we produced was validated by a responsible group. Eventually all our documents, both written and schematic, had to be accepted through the faculty council and also the assembly of department heads.

- We presented the program two or three times to the assemblé facultaire and we also sent it to the heads of departments, asking them to have special department assemblies to critique the written report. Likewise, the dean sent "Le programme des études" to each department head. As I recall, the process went from the school executive, namely, the deans and vice-deans and the faculty council, which is composed of 14 persons elected, all of whom received the same document, then to the heads of departments, and then to the general assembly of faculty.

Opposition at Sherbrooke to such broad-scale change, as at Hawaii, also came principally from basic scientists who feared being disempowered by problem-based teaching and learning. Five years after the fact, some still question both the new pedagogy's means, in suppressing department- and discipline-based teaching, and ends, in graduating, as the critics perceive them, mere medical technicians.

- [In committee] our biggest difficulty . . . was with the medical biologists. Their difficulty was in seeing that they would be losing hours, losing lecture time, that sort of thing. Our solution was to give them 2 full months at the beginning of the program, 2 full months for a medical biology unit. We said, "Okay, we will compromise." We said to them, "You take the first semester of the first year, entirely, except for the last 3 weeks, which we need for clinical immersion." But they did not push their opposition, and so we all have moved ahead. You see, it was difficult for them. They thought they were losing parts of the curriculum. Keep in mind that the basic sciences are not that strong anyway. They really only have the first year because of the organ systems organization of the second and third year. The basic scientists warned that research would suffer under the new program, that the practice plan would go into bankruptcy, and that the residency program would suffer. [I: Was there any merit in their arguments?] No, not at all. Since the new program has come into effect, research money has risen from $11 to $20 million, practice plan income has risen by 7 to 10% per annum, and our residency programs are now better, in fact. As for support, it came from the people who were learning new skills, because at the same time we were instituting a faculty development program. In the last 5 years since the program began, 40% of our faculty have undergone 100 hours of faculty development in 3-hour sessions. I would say that at the beginning in 1987, 30% of our faculty were in favor of the new program. With more and more experience in the program, that percentage has risen sharply.

- We were presented all at once with the change. It was not a public process at first. [I: And when it became public?] I would say that 80 to 90% of the faculty were against problem-based learning and so forth. But participation then gradually created agreement. Most faculty went through the training sessions that we had. In these sessions we were asked why we thought we were here. Was it to teach or was it to make students learn? And can they learn more effectively with newer methods? This was in 1985–1986. I was strongly impressed by this. We said, "Damn it, that is true." But at the same time, the unconvinced said, "Let us leave the door open a little, let us be careful." Still, with the GPEP recommendations published by then, we realized that we were on the right track. Within 1 or 2 years, half of our faculty members were participating in the new program enthusiastically. By now I would say 95% are cooperating readily. But there is still the problem of faculty feeling used without being heard. [I: Is this a significant problem?] I cannot tell yet. In my 15– to 20–person group, I would say that more than five are very critical of this. Let me say that among the basic scientists, we see the MD as more than just giving aspirin. We are more likely to be dissatisfied with what is being done than the clinical people.

[I: What are your deepest reservations about the new curriculum?] One is the existence of departments. They tend to disintegrate in this method. In the new curriculum, there is no direct accountability because departments are not involved. Eventually the departments will lose a great deal. Second, the primary thing in an MD program is to teach well and to learn well. But to continue to have professors who teach well and who teach for tomorrow, the departments and the disciplines must survive and continue to attract the people who will eventually replace us as teachers. At places like Harvard, Washington University, McGill, Barcelona, the Sorbonne, Padova, there are faculties with a tradition of producing teachers as well as practitioners of medicine. From my class, the class of 1960–1961, there are now 20 professors scattered throughout the world. How many professors will come from Sherbrooke? The raw material is here, but it comes into a technology of application. If application is all that you learn while you are in medical school, there is no time to recoup later, because soon enough there is a job, a family, taxes to pay, and so forth. Therefore, my fear is that we will have two kinds of medical schools and medical faculties. I am afraid that we are coming to this. And with the inbreeding at Sherbrooke and the way that we recruit faculty from among our own students, the tendency is even stronger.

CHAPTER 6

Implementation

In curriculum as in carpentry, the time comes to put the boat in the water, the plan into practice, to concede in some fashion, with the innovators at Sherbrooke, that,

> If we had prepared any more, then we would have stopped. You see, if you do not start, then you will not do it. You must make a decision and go forward. In retrospect, you may say many things, but that is only retrospect. For example, if we had known what would be required of us, we might not have tried it. But we needed to do it, and we were confident. Plus there was already a lot of work done and many people were ready to change. My experience is that if you think too much, you stand still.

This is when implementation begins. Yet, planners in complex institutions like medical schools can never design with complete enough knowledge nor implement with complete enough authority to have projects turn out completely as envisioned. Consequences always come intended and unintended, and both sorts constitute outcomes.

At Mercer, where the 1982 charter class tested out the new curriculum, a less ponderous first year was in place by 1984 and so on for successive years. Adjustments, readily made at such an early point in so small a program, aimed to adapt design concept to internal and external reality, to teaching practice as it unfolded, and to program accreditation criteria as these impinged on the curriculum. Eased by the school's improving financial picture, adjustments included more precisely locating basic- and behavioral-sciences instruction, adding a phase on infectious diseases, redefining learning goals and evaluation procedures, and adapting curriculum content to board certification. As it would at Case Western Reserve, a high failure rate on the boards caught people's attention at Mercer and, as McMaster would too, the school added objective measures of student performance.

- The curriculum was designed already when we came here [in 1982]. It was in the first year of implementation when Hockman, Volpe, and I took it over and made it into our own flavor. So there was a far bigger change between year 0 and year 2 in 1984 than there has been since year 2 to the present. With the charter class, everything was a new experience for us. But by the third class we knew pretty much what we wanted from the freshman year in the basic-science parts. Then, with each subsequent year, we knew, respectively, what we pretty much wanted from the second, the third, and the fourth years and made the corresponding changes. The biggest changes have included finding a niche for the behavioral sciences, putting the basic sciences in specific phases of the program rather than throughout it, figuring the difference between what the national boards want and what we want, and adding a phase in infectious diseases because microbiology turned out weak in the first years. But we have also had to define learning objectives for the first two phases. These were defined by the old guys but then we had to redefine them. On the one hand, Warner had defined a very theoretical system of teaching from the molecular to the cellular to the cell tissue and higher levels. We went on to specify these further in definite cases. On the other hand, we instituted big changes in evaluation. Warner was pedagogically good but very impractical. His major evaluation was the tutorial evaluation. He took it from Kansas, the quarterly profile exam. It was a very subjective system. With Waddell Barnes from Harvard, Hockman from Illinois, and me from Michigan State, there was more appreciation for cognitive evaluation. We thought that otherwise students would do poorly on the national boards. After all, half of the charter class failed the boards on the first try. We thought that they had been set up to fail. So we created an evaluation system in three parts: tutorial evaluation, oral examination, and multidisciplinary examination. Dick Menninger defined the guidelines.

- Through the early 1990s, the financial picture improved. State grant aid and capitation went up, and from 24 students we moved to 49 at present. All are Georgians, all from the state. We get $10,000 per capita per year plus the grants. This has been a very big help in improving the financial picture. Likewise since 1985, the medical center has been very supportive of graduate medical education. It was then that they recognized that the community teaching hospital would be a thing of the past and that you had to bring in qualified graduate faculty. Their investment in medical education then increased 10 to 15% a year measured by education outlays. For many of the faculty people that they brought in, we trade off reimbursements. Total resources available for medical education are now $24 million per annum. Of that the state furnishes one-third, the university one-third, and the Medical Center of Central Georgia one-third. The latter pays for all graduate medical education at Mercer through direct support of the faculty involved. The center's one-third does not flow through the dean's budget, however, but they do provide documents that go into our LCME report. Our total budget puts us in the lower 15% of U.S. medical schools in terms of revenue. We have little endowment after all. We need a Bowman Gray to fund us. [At first] finances were very tough, very tight. When I came, the state was putting in about $4.5 million a year. It is now up to $8 million including capitation and state grants. [I: Who brought that about?] I did, working with the university vice president for government relations, John Mitchell.

Outcome closely reflects intention at Mercer because innovation came with the new school's founding; because deans appropriate to the school's changing needs over a decade's operation were found; and because Mercer's small size precluded basic-science departments, the loci of turf-based instruction at larger schools and natural antagonists of problem-based teaching and learning. Tellingly, department organization now stands as the major barrier to implementing innovation in the clinical years.

- The biggest, most important decision ever taken here, which is directly related to our success, was not to allow the basic scientists to have departments. We meet as a division of basic science, anatomists, physiologists, everyone. It is fun to watch the conflicts as much as anything else. There is loose organization by disciplinary groups to evaluate our students, but everyone knows that in curriculum matters a microbiologist is not just a microbiologist here at Mercer. The barrier of department lines is the single greatest barrier to implementing effective problem-based programs in the country. This is why at Michigan State in the track two committee, department chairs were not admitted. Right now, the barrier to innovation in the clinical years is precisely what the chairs represent. We know how problem-based learning works and how it would work in the clinical years. We know how to do it. The only obstacle is the organization, what the clinical chairs represent in terms of stratification of the institution, therefore stratification of the curriculum. You cannot have problem-based learning and have disciplinary-political lines in the way.

When implementation falls short at Mercer, it is viewed more as unfinished business than as failure, as the periodic need to adapt concept, not abandon it, to reality inside and outside the school.

- We have been able as much as anyone to integrate problem-based medical education longitudinally, but we are not there yet. We still need to improve in interdisciplinary ways. The multidisciplinary exam is still multidisciplinary, not interdisciplinary. The microbiologists, the anatomists, the physiologists, still submit their own questions. We are trying to find ways to enrich the quality of interdisciplinary approaches here and to reward it. We are working along the lines of writing interdisciplinary questions. There is a related need for us to improve oral examinations. Some faculty have become complacent in oral examinations. So it goes back to basics, to revitalization and revival at the grass roots, to bring original purpose and program ownership back to the tutors and the phase coordinators. We need a revival.

Hawaii's implementation, just under way, is more complicated than Mercer's, because it did not begin from scratch; because the innovation intends to reach, more radically, across all 4, including the 2 clinical, years; and because Hawaii's commanding dean-entrepreneur has made a remarkable end run not just around departments but around academic organization per se.

- To emphasize programs instead of departments . . . we are trying to congregate all the basic science departments into one biomedical program [and] we are changing the way students carry out their activities. We want them not to follow the faculty but to follow the patients. We want them to bump up against various disciplines as they follow the patients. We have been talking about this following-the-patient idea for a long time. [I: Who's we?] Myself, Max Botticelli in the department of medicine, and Ralph Hale. But there is something else too that faculty has not fully comprehended yet. My problem with universities is that they are . . . structured to prevent change. My view is that a medical school should lead change, not follow it. Therefore the school must be nimble, flexible, and communicate well at all levels so that rumors do not get out of hand and prevent change. So only after we changed to problem-based learning, I proposed refocusing organizationally from departments to programs. I did this after the change because I did not want to scare the hell out of faculty by doing too much too fast. To put it simply, I redefined the role of the associate deans! I moved them to the side of the organizational chart, to the vertical column, and said, "The deans of education, research, service are just the keepers of the mission . . . you facilitate that mission across all the programs of the school." All program directors answer to the dean without anyone, including associate deans, in between to filter information. The MD program, for example, is only one of 25 programs at the medical school. The departments may have their own programs, for example, a residency in internal medicine or a PhD in anatomy, and serve as resource units to all other programs. In this respect the department chairs become resource managers to the school's various programs.

But where I put the money is into the program directors, not into the department chairs! Then, we carry on an entrepreneurial game. I promote a buy-and-sell relationship between the directors and the chairs. Say, for example, that the MD program needs three tutors. It takes 10% of a faculty member's time to be a unit tutor, so for a salary of $50,000 a year that would be $5,000. The MD program director says, I am buying these tutors, does any chair want to sell me three tutors? If no chair sells the director a tutor, the rules are that the director can go outside the school, into the university or into any other university. No one can block the process. I tell the chairs, "Buy all three and then go out and recruit them." I say, "Buy them for $2,500 and sell them for $5,000."

I have the program directors directly under me and I have the chairs servicing the programs. It is improving communication. It has gotten people's attention. The flexibility in this is inherent. Say we have an HIV residency program. What if tomorrow there is an AIDS vaccine? We just erase the program and, when a new disaster arises, I just add a program! [I: Where is the funding for these?] Out of my office. I am the principal investigator for most schoolwide programs and I look for funding anywhere I can get it, from the public, the legislature, foundations, private individuals. My whole life has been as an entrepreneur. I tell the program directors, "Look, I am ultimately responsible for how the money is spent and you are responsible for getting the money." And I can change a director overnight, because it is not a regular faculty-approved appointment as an associate dean would be. I have discovered that there are two things about change. There is change inside the school, which I have been describing to you, and change outside the school. My view is, do not fight the bureaucracy because it is there to protect the status quo. Instead just starve it and create a new one to protect the change. Thus for the Kellogg grant, for example, I developed a nonprofit corporation to fit the program, and I am the chairman of the board. The board includes the dean of the college of health sciences, the provost of the community colleges, the director of the state department of health, and the directors and board members of each of the participating clinics. The board numerically favors the communities! The point is, do not engage the bureaucracy in a tug-of-war.

Nevertheless, charismatic or command-style leadership in academic institutions, even in those that afford faculty so little voice, always reaches a limit, in part because it awakens, if not emboldens, that voice.

- The problem has always been with raising your voice and being heard. [I: In governance bodies?] I do not even know what the official name of that body is here. There is some sort of faculty governance committee that is supposed to function like a faculty senate, but it has no real powers. [I: Isn't there a curriculum committee under the faculty?] It was virtually inactive until recently. [I: Did it come to life with the change?] Yes, in part, and this has had to do with some new faculty leadership. In the last governance meeting called by faculty, it was debated whether we should continue or expand the six-E program. [I: Six-E?] It means "six experimental" and it is a program in the third year, which instead of having clerkship rotations and having students see all types of patients along the route, gets them to follow patients all the way from the beginning to the end. This is the first year of the six-E program and it takes six to 10 students a year. If it proves acceptable, it might take up to 50% percent of our students . . . eventually the entire class. [But] many clinical faculty do not agree with it philosophically. They say if it ain't broke don't fix it.

If authority may be observed as the probability that a directive will be followed, then the collegial authority known for centuries inside universities gives and follows directions by consensus more than command, thus in a way very different from either charismatic or bureaucratic authority. For all its innova-

tive nature, then, the change at Hawaii is more person- than institution-embodied and thus less stable or predictable in outcome.

- We continue to implement change, but the problem is
  really in communication. Members of the MD committee
  do not do a good job communicating with faculty. Faculty in
  turn worry that this body is making decisions that are out
  of touch not only with school but also with the community.
  We are so decentralized as an academic health center that
  communication will make or break us. We are in 11 different hospitals in this city alone! The building that we are in
  now is the biomedical research building, not the medical
  school. This is only the research part of the medical school.
  The rest is out there in many places. There are two things
  that offer a solution to this. First, an E-mail system across
  all platforms including DOS [disk operating system], Mac-
  intosh, and so forth. Second, we are developing an interactive video system to be placed in every operational site, every hospital, wherever we have students and residents, so
  that grand rounds can be held without everyone having to
  move and consulting can be conducted without consultants
  having to move. The system is designed both for education
  and for patient services.
- The process on paper looks extremely good, but in fact it
  does not use faculty as resource people as effectively as it
  could. Students do not always seek the counsel of faculty,
  and faculty are not always as receptive to students as they
  might be. Before problem-based learning, there was a rigid
  schedule in place way in advance. Now it is more hit-or-
  miss. We need a better way to use faculty resource people.
  This is the weakness of our program to date if there is one.
  As for the community medicine part, it is happening but
  there are rough edges. There is a group of students who do
  not think that they need it. They think that the hospice rotation, for example, is not a doctor's business. They think
  that it is not up to the doctor to deal with death and dying.
  They think that dying should be turfed out to someone
  else. This year's class is better on the subject, however. I

think that we have been indoctrinating students much better recently and that we have improved the experience.

- In the problem-based learning process the main items that they hit initially are anatomy, physiology, and pathophysiology. But because of the limitation of time there is only cursory exposure to pharmacology, biochemistry, and microbiology. The strong positives for problem-based learning are self-learning, problem solving, and less stress because students are not constantly taking exams. I personally enjoy tutoring and like it more than lecturing. My concern is that while the top half of students do as well or better than in the traditional system, the bottom half really struggles, particularly those with minimal science background. They need a lot of discipline to fill in the gaps. It is not a very efficient form of learning. Given unlimited time it would be a great system, but given limited time, there are problems. Thus I suppose we have exchanged information overload for information gaps. It is the swing of the pendulum. The first class to go through with problem-based learning, which is the present fourth-year class, was pretty much a disaster and did rather poorly on the national boards. The second was average. The third class is coming up now. We will have to see.

My concern is the nonsystemic way of learning in the problem-based approach. [I: Can you learn systemically inside problem-based learning? Will students have to do it on their own to fill in the gaps? Do they do that?] In some ways, yes, because they have to prepare for the boards. They have a 9–week block to prepare for the boards. Because of my concern about this, for that last traditional class of 1990, I had my faculty write a series of syllabi which were actually their written-up lecture notes. We had the option to give lectures but we chose not to. Instead for the class of 1990 we gave ten conferences that were basically lectures. They then took our exams the usual way and they did very well. And on the national boards they did just as well as previously, maybe even a little better. Therefore we felt confident that we had a system that could help the students even with problem-based learning coming. It was a combination of syllabi and exams and a computer bank of questions.

Even clinician colleagues, for example, have bridled at the dean's effort to streamline formerly quite autonomous departments' clinical instruction at Hawaii.

- [The dean's] thinking began with the idea of changing training in the clinical years. To do this, he knew that he needed to change the first 2 years, and of course he is exactly right. The clinical departments at Hawaii have traditionally been very autonomous. [I: How does the dean want to change the clinical years?] From his point of view, there are two things. First, have primary care integrated across the whole curriculum of the third year. Second, create more outpatient experience for students. The emphasis on primary care is built around the McMaster concept of streamlining the clinical departments. There was in fact a lot of overlap among these departments here and a corresponding need for coordination, for example, between the departments of medicine and of surgery in treating the subject of ulcers. So the dean brought these departments together to decide what students needed to know and to recognize how much overlap there was. Everyone agreed that things could be improved. The solution to this is to integrate the clerkships, and many recognized the need for this. It is very much in line with attacking the concept of teaching baby specialists. As for giving students more outpatient experience, there are differences among the clinical departments. The pediatricians actually handle patients on an inpatient basis even though it is mostly acute care at the Kapiolani Children's Hospital. Medicine and surgery, which are at Queen's hospital, tend to be more outpatient. So pediatrics was inpatient but a better teaching environment, while medicine and surgery were outpatient but a worse teaching environment. The dean began to correct this and was the central author of the MD program committee, which he put in charge of the entire clinical curriculum. To date it is still in collision with the tradition of autonomy of the existing clinical departments here.

New Mexico's 1970s implementation was easier than Hawaii's 1980s effort because it focused only on the first two years and was designed down one column, as a protected track, not across-the-board. As near optimal as a concept-to-application scenario may be, despite its own guinea-pig class's high failure rate on the boards, changes were phased in gradually by a small, informal, foundation-funded, dean-supported faculty group.

- We started with 10 students in 1979 and went to 20 students very soon thereafter, using a Kellogg Foundation grant. It has remained at about 20 since then. We did not change the third year at all, but the first 2 years were changed considerably. When the first class in the primary-class curriculum took part one of the national boards, it was clear that they did not know the humerus from the femur. It was clear that they needed some morphology. With this feedback, changes were introduced in the new curriculum. Some of the earlier observations were also that primary-care curriculum students were entering clerkships in the third year more articulate and more communicative than traditional-track students, although the differences disappeared entering the second year of clerkships. Thus the traditional kids caught up. . . . [I: Any problems at first?] Some said that it took too much teaching time from preclinical faculty . . . that, before, you could take all 73 students in an entering class and give them one lecture, whereas now you had to put much more effort into tutorials for small groups of students. At first, people really had no idea of what would happen. They wondered if students would pass the boards, for example. Clinicians wondered if the students would be qualified when they came into their rotations third year. But these concerns evaporated over time.

Implementers at New Mexico had time to run the experiment, learn from experience, and adapt. Early innovators, they implemented a plan in the 1970s with little record to go on, and, over the 1980s, periodically realigned intent by outcome, the prerogative of unhurried inventors left more or less to their own devices.

- There have been modifications in student performance evaluation, first of all. For example, in 1981 a report was issued on our students' performance on the national boards' part one and on their deficiency in anatomy. There have also been evaluations that brought changes in how we teach student–patient interactions and in our problem-based learning format. We have sought more exposure to the basic sciences of medicine, for example, and in problem-based learning we have sought more effective problems with which to get across basic principles. From a methodological point of view, the real problem in our evaluation, however, is that we ain't got no control group, in the scientific sense. There is no virginal traditional track as in 1978 any longer, and no virginal primary-care track as in 1978. Without real experimental method and no real controls, our evaluations end up showing different shades of gray. It is hard to write scientific papers on these data for lack of controls.

    Each department has participated to a degree. With the initial grant from Kellogg, there was money available to stimulate the departments. As time went on, some faculty, naturally, got more heavily involved. Then, some got grants and reduced their time in the program and others increased their participation. One of our underlying goals here is that we attempt within the faculty, or within the departments, to create a division of labor related to individual interests. For example, for some clinical faculty, their talent may be in patient care, for others, it may be in their research contribution, and so we reduce patient care time. As I see it, the two common threads that hold the institution together here are education and the parking problem. [I: Did the administration support the new program?] Yes, both in terms of being persuaded that as an academic institution we need to undertake experiments and in terms of fiscal allocation. After the Kellogg grant ended, for example, the question was how to replace those moneys, for example, how to continue support for students' 4–month preceptorials, how to support the departments and the instructors involved with these. I found various means to accomplish these ends. I have tried to be a constructive cynic over the years of the primary-care curriculum here. I have suggested from time to time that a lecture might not be immoral. My method is to stand away from people who want to accomplish something, in other words to not get in their way. [I: What went well, not well in these years?] Well is that the administration and faculty were prepared to look at and to evaluate what was being done and to identify things that gave new ideas for both the primary-care and traditional tracks. We keep looking at performance and modifying things. Not so well, is that at times there has been a drawing in of wagons, of primary-care curriculum faculty and students against traditional-track faculty and students and vice versa. At times, collegiality has been very low.

* The group worked well together. We had a good staff. There was lots of camaraderie. We found out about the McMaster program. We learned a lot of things in that period. We learned to interact with faculty. Most of them, of course, were friends. We developed credibility over the years. Even the chair of radiology, who before had shot down every idea I had said, said, "Great Scot! Go for it!" Also, we had to bribe everyone, except the chair of orthopedics. We really hurt his feelings by not funding him right at the start. But we filled it in later. There were lots of conflicts of personality, just personality stuff. As I see it, Arthur's style is to do it yesterday and mine is to drag my feet. But without this combination we would not have gotten anywhere.

In the 1990s, however, change at New Mexico has become more complicated, and outcome less assured, as, foundation-driven again, some of the same innovators now seek to integrate two long-separated experimental and traditional tracks. Still, strong continuities favor the latest installment of ongoing experiment at New Mexico.

* [I: What brought on the present effort to integrate the two curricula?] First, in reading the Robert Wood Johnson

Foundation proposal several years ago, we knew that, to get support, the curriculum had to benefit all students, that there could be no tracks. This pushed us to integrate. Second, a strategic plan of the curriculum committee, I think it was in 1987–1988, recommended keeping the two tracks but doing more ambulatory-care teaching. Third, the LCME [Liaison Committee on Medical Education] had us look at their concerns after the recent cycle. We instituted a self-study. But the primary catalyst was the Robert Wood Johnson Foundation proposal. We would not have moved as quickly to integrate the 2 tracks without the Robert Wood Johnson Foundation program. [I: Would it be possible to generalize the primary-care curriculum track?] Yes, perhaps, but there is just too much jealousy on this campus, too much distrust of those of us for whom the primary-care curriculum has been very good. But there is a deeper problem, a problem with respect to paradigm. We are trying to create a significant paradigm shift in education here. And some of our faculty even now are resisting it. One department chair two weeks ago said that the tutorials are like a videotape to him. After 14 years, this is how much he understands the primary-care curriculum program. Faculty is split, really, in terms of belief and trust in students to learn on their own. I would say half or more of the basic scientists do not trust students in this way and the clinicians couldn't give a damn really.

[Are you optimistic about the process of integrating the traditional- and primary-care curriculum tracks? What are the best- and worst-case scenarios in the next 3 to 4 years?] In the best case, it goes smoothly; in the worst, faculty revolt and say hell no. [I: How would such a faculty revolt look?] Well, a group of however many faculty submit a letter to the dean to vote to proceed to do away with the primary-care curriculum, to do just the conventional curriculum as it exists. It would take 51% of the faculty. [I: What would increase the likelihood of this?] Well, they would rally their allies and try to keep it quiet. They would have to cut down on their bitching and make sure that the faculty vote on this in faculty meeting, because the dean would resist it at all costs. But I think in general the faculty is smarter than to try to do this. They know that New Mexico would then move back to the mediocre level of medical schools. Some schools are already asking me, "Are you dropping problem-based learning?" In fact, even the guys going to NIH [National Institutes of Health], the basic scientists applying for grants, benefit from our reputation, because people have heard about problem-based learning at the University of New Mexico. And they are more likely to be funded being at a place with a reputation for doing interesting stuff.

• [The recent effort] continues to refocus faculty on medical student education. The original concept was that medical school faculty, or some faculty, especially in the basic-science departments, were becoming very, very pro forma. They were teaching the same thing year after year. What is happening now has especially affected the clinical department faculty, both in terms of the first 2 years' basic-science and the second 2 years. And we have had some optimal results, some really collegial results, between basic science and clinical faculty based on educational practices that have spawned common research questions. These come as a result of getting them together to discuss educational matters that bridge areas that are otherwise not neatly bridged. People began saying, "Well, maybe ... well, let's see" and that sort of thing. When people discuss the neural sciences over the course of a 4–year program, there can be spin-offs that are directly related to research or patient care, or that give basic scientists the means to illustrate basic principles in a way that is more interesting to students than the more pedantic approach.

Minnesota, in its own up-from-the-bottom, at-the-margin, individually sponsored, unwritten way, has closely joined intent and outcome, especially in integrating the basic and clinical sciences since the mid-1980s. Its success in this is due, however, to the determination of only a very few innovators.

• There have been a number of positive things not always written down. First, I would guess that almost half the course directors for the first year now are clinical faculty. Just this fact means that the basic science council is no longer an exclusive club of PhDs. These clinicians, however, are very research oriented. Second, we have the clinical correlations that Kaplan runs. He is a believer in basic science and clinical integration. Kaplan has chosen faculty in basic science and clinical medicine to participate together. Often there is a patient there, too, during correlations. [I: Has he been supported by the basic-science departments in his efforts?] He would say no. [I: Who wants, who does not want him to succeed?] The course directors and the educational policy committee will give him nonfinancial support for correlations in the first year. The course directors were skeptical at first, but now he is one of the guys. They were worried about simple-minded cases, but Kaplan has done a very good job at it, for example, in the biochemistry course with Livingston. [I: Are there correlations in all the basic-science courses?] Not as a separate entity. But Kaplan has succeeded in biochemistry. Correlations are not part of the core, not part of the evaluation in this course, but more and more faculty are saying informally to students that you are responsible for the correlations, even though it is not a rule. [I: The norm at Minnesota?] That's the point! The unsaid, unspoken, unwritten often works better. [I: Any other things in the first year?] Yes, in the spring and summer there are eight lectures on medical ethics. [I: Are these effective?] Yes, a small group of us can do it. Kaplan, our ethicist, is very much sought after, a real clinical presence in the first year. Then too, there is what we used to call "Return to Basic Science," which had some merit, but which students were not open to in the fourth year. They all had to come in for 2 weeks from all over the place, from all over the city and state, and they were unhappy about this. [I: Is there any functional equivalent to it now?] Yes, the second unit of pathophysiology has reproduced it. It has a strong basic-science content.

At Case Western Reserve over the same period, there has been little innovation to implement since discipline-based departments there, in contrast to an earlier time, have come to define the educational agenda. Consistent with the school's mounting status anxiety over the 1980s, an agenda so defined has focused less on predoctoral education—neither on innovative, for example, epidemiologic, content nor on problem-based teaching and learning methods—than on postdoctoral studies.

- My impression is that our primary concerns have been how facts can be transmitted more effectively and how the use of these facts can be taught more effectively, for example, in problem-based learning. [I: Is this bad?] No, not at all. [I: But it misses something?] Yes, it misses a certain evangelical feature of the school, and, oddly enough, it does not focus really scientific attention on what our practice should consist of. Its primary failure lies in not examining our practice, for example, in entirely missing the grave epidemiological side to contemporary medical practice. You see, the medical school is saddled with department chairs who are more preoccupied with postdoctoral fellows and with residents than with medical students. Thus at Lakeside Hospital last year, the real crisis was that we failed to fill all our internships, not that 22% of medical students failed part one of the national boards. There is also the problem that people come here to teach for 4 years and then go elsewhere. [I: Would any of the 1952–type reforms address these problems?] I think so. The idea of a "blast" physician recognizes the fact that you cannot turn out a finished product. You only have them for 4 years. It is a structural problem. But training such physicians requires faculty time and the academic economy nowadays apparently dictates that teaching be done with less expenditure of faculty time. One of the shocking things to me is that the committee on medical education now has closed meetings and excludes spectators like myself. Another change in recent years is that some of the basic-science chairs now want to teach straight anatomy and biochemistry and so forth, rather than organ systems. This has not been brought up in any general faculty meeting, which now are little-attended in any case.

Consistent with how it was designed at Dartmouth, the school's recent outpatient clerkship program has been implemented by a nimble administrator's end run around otherwise preoccupied department chairs. To the extent that change occurs more by individual than institutional effort, outcome remains as iffy as at Dartmouth or at Minnesota.

- When we announced at the [1989] AAMC [American Association of Medical Colleges] meeting that 25% of our clerkships were outpatient, everyone was amazed. But our chairs were pissed because students in outpatient settings slowed them down. [When one chair] asked who was going to pay for this, I said, "You agreed to, remember?" It was a big shock to him. Obviously he had not taken it seriously. The chairs were all looking at the power issues, at their share in the total number of weeks, and not the implications of outpatient settings for student education and the cost of it. We did this in August 1989. When the LCME made outpatient clerkship mandatory in the late 1980s and the AAMC changed it from a should to a must in 1990, I felt that my neck was saved, because this all happened a year or two after we did it at Dartmouth. So the big change in clerkships here in Dartmouth came about just because of a frustrated dean and a very simplistic calendar change issue. After that I just did my own thing! The clerkship coordinator for surgery, now a convert to the community-based component, came to me shortly after the change and asked, "Where is that dictum that says that 25% of the clerkships needs to be in a primary care setting?" I said, "There isn't any! We just set it up ourselves!" He was quite surprised, but by then he was on board and he is now a big proponent of the 25% system.

Dartmouth's current institutionwide review of predoctoral studies generates only guarded optimism among those familiar with the school's overwhelmingly content-based education legacy.

- [I: What will the curriculum look like in 5 years?] Very similar to now, I would guess. My one hope is, if nothing else, to bang heads of the faculty enough to decrease content overload in courses. I am not necessarily a big proponent of problem-based learning, even though it may be better than some techniques. In research that I have done here, I found four teachers who in front of 70 to 90 students could produce significant interaction in a lecture course and were able to conduct actual conversations regularly with students in lecture. Therefore I think that, if there are not enough resources for problem-based learning, this kind of contact can be done other ways. [I: So what will change?] Maybe the look of the diagrams of classes, but I will be very surprised if we succeed in putting clerkship experience into the first year. Personally . . . I think the system needs to be totally changed. I think that science needs to be learned in clinical settings. I would put them into patient-care settings from the start, then give them science courses concurrently. I am very radical. The faculty is so afraid here that a student will kill or mutilate some patient.

The change implemented top-down over the 1980s at Harvard, in a pedagogical experiment that required willing faculty and an attentive dean, comes as close as any to realizing its intent.

- Only 2 years into the new program, many faculty were calling for a thorough evaluation of the New Pathway. So the dean had the department of anatomy, which was teaching two courses, standard and experimental, come before the other basic-science departments, saying "We can only teach one course. It is too expensive to teach two. So we will go with the experimental course." He did this after only 2 years of experimentation! So then the rest of the faculty did not want to teach two courses either, experimental and standard, at which point you never saw so many faculty who had been against the experimental method sell out so quickly and accept the New Pathway! The dean was very skillful. Tosteson made it happen and most of the students are happier with the new curriculum now. I have sat in endless curriculum committee meetings where, if the dean had ever put it up to a closed ballot, he would have lost the New Pathway. Instead, he would go to the meetings himself and the deal would pass because faculty did not have the balls to oppose him. So Tosteson made it happen here. I remember when Douglas Bond was dean at Case Western, he too knew how to get things done. For example, he knew that the major opponent to the new curriculum then was the chair of the department of obstetrics. So he made sure to join him at tea one day before the discussion of his proposals. He sat right next to him. Then, as the meeting got under way, he asked everyone to state their views around in a circle, so that his major opponent had the last comment. He was 30th to speak. He gave up and held his tongue. After the meeting Bond gave him another ten thousand square feet for the department!

New Pathway proponents nevertheless find fault in how watered down the centerpiece patient–doctor course soon became and in how little innovation took place in critical content areas like epidemiology.

- In its first implementation the patient–doctor course was highly successful, partly because its failures helped it succeed. Both students and faculty were incredibly engaged in the course and they criticized it well. I believe that that level of engagement is part of what made them learn. Our evaluation suggests that it was incredibly effective, that it made a measurable difference. But 3 to 4 years into the new program, the course was changed and the socialization changed with it. The course was then no longer a continuous unbroken theme in the curriculum with the same faculty over 3 years. Content has been drastically watered down since then. It has narrowed its focus to something almost antiintellectual. This is not the way it was early on when, if anything, there was too much intellectual content and it was too complicated. Now the course is molded from the top down and it has been devalued of serious content.
- The New Pathway was a big change in the system . . . a step forward, yes. But at Harvard we never added the issues that they did at Johns Hopkins, namely, medical education related to public need. Our thrust was instead to improve the intellectual quality of learning here. We have never thought of our school as one that prepared family-care or primary-care physicians particularly [because] here we are fascinated with molecular biology, with its precise eloquent models and investigations, and with its findings.

We think that we are getting closer and closer to the meaning of life in this way. Thus even if I can show that social buffers, social relationships, protect against mortality, for example, it can never be as clearly shown how. The intervening mechanisms remain vague, unlike prescribing insulin for diabetes. I do not know how to write prescriptions for making friends. So it is still the hard sciences that attract students, the big problems in molecular biology. The other sciences, they are told, are touchy-feely. Most do not understand a thing about epidemiology, for example. One thing that would make a difference is the idea that David Sackett at McMaster has to introduce clinical epidemiology into the clinical years by teaching around cases. The likelihood of students paying attention to social factors and taking them seriously is increased if you see that patient as a member of an occupational or ethnic group. It is not enough to teach the stuff just the first year. Epidemiology needs integrating into the clinical years. Therefore we need to educate the clinical faculty in particular. By this time the basic scientists are really through with the students.

It would also make a big difference if from the dean on down a medical school took the message of population-based medicine as an explicit guideline to policy. To tell students the day that they arrive that population-based medicine is important would make a big difference. Instead our dean greets students in the first class meeting by saying, "Half the things you learn will be outdated by the time you are practicing." He tells them what an interesting time it is to be entering medicine. What he should say instead, I think, is that a third of the population is left out of health care and remains uncared for. He should say, "Do something about it." ... If the administration really believed what it says about the population-based sciences, it would have to reexamine our mission and either change to more primary care or deliberately justify the specialist proportion of our graduates. In other words, it would have to make conscious its reasons for that proportion.

University of California, San Francisco (UCSF), prodded by the dean, aided by a new admissions policy, and instructed by a talented pedagogue, implemented specific changes that have very effectively reinvolved the basic scientists in teaching and learning, neglecting which they had to some extent precipitated a student revolt in the mid-1980s. The clinicians at UCSF have yet to be brought into predoctoral instruction as effectively as they have been at Minnesota.

- We have made a complete turnaround in the last decade with respect to our educational mission. The basic scientists here now love to teach. And the students are very satisfied with this part of the curriculum. We have succeeded less well in the clinical areas. It is harder to bring the clinicians into the education mission of the school because the clinicians are such a diffuse group. There are so many rungs. It is like the Chinese Communist Party. As you go further and further into it, it gets more and more diffuse. It goes right into the market place!

Thus if outcome reflects intent in basic sciences instruction at UCSF, it clearly does not do so in the clinical arena, in large part because of the clinicians' growing need, as elsewhere, to support themselves.

- The clinical departments have to be restructured. This would be difficult but not impossible. One of the things we tried was having the education policy and curriculum committee put very stringent requirements on the clinical departments concerning what the goals were for clinical clerkships. I wanted our students to do passbooks to help establish exactly what they had experienced. In the process we discovered that few students had ever done a pelvic examination! And many were never observed doing a physical exam. After 2 years of residency, our students often told us that it was their clinical skills that were weakest: history taking, physical exam, and so forth. As a result, our current number one problem is the fractive line between the basic and clinical years. It is still very apparent. It really goes back to the problem of the research institute in the Humboltian University, which was never resolved, but we are better here than most. . . . The problem is the rigidity of the clinical departments in their inability to switch to better teaching methods and more contact time with students. Recently, in fact, contact time has decreased, not increased, because of the demands on clinicians to support themselves. If Clinton succeeds in putting caps on all payments, it will be very rough on the medical schools.

The clinical instruction of predoctoral students is inhibited at UCSF by the twin forces of preadmissions patient diagnosis in teaching hospitals and, as at Harvard, the super-specialization of instructors.

- There are problems with procedures and with specialization. Virtually every patient is subject now to an enormous number of procedures. Patients come in almost entirely diagnosed with the data in hand. For students this is not interesting. The learning potential in seeing patients is thus enormously decreased. Most patients are there for only a few days, rarely more than 6 days, and so medical students have little time to contemplate and to do step-wise thinking. We need to get students into outpatient settings or doctors' offices. The problem is space . . . for these settings and the time, which amounts to money, for working with ambulatory patients. A visit combined with teaching can take an hour instead of 10 minutes. The problem is that students are overexposed to the importance of procedures at the expense of primary-care diagnosis, at the expense of smelling, tasting, looking. We also have super-specialization here at the university hospital. . . . You have to have this sort of specialization in bone marrow transplant work for leukemia, for example. But at the same time it does not make sense to teach medical students on these services. Medical students who are thus exposed only to subspecialties do not know how to take a history and they are weak in physical examination and differential diagnoses.

Regrettably, tough yet solvable problems in clinical instruction may be rendered unsolvable by the overarching issues, nowhere as severe as at UCSF, of space and department organization.

- So the changes worked in the basic sciences but less in the clinical sciences. Even so what we accomplished is now under stress because of space and financial problems.
- Let me tell you two things that I undertook [unsuccessfully]. First . . . the state of California is mandating that 50% of graduates of our medical schools go into primary care. So I tried but failed to make a primary-care department. I tried to combine family and community medicine with general internal medicine and general pediatrics. I wanted to make family care a real specialty. I would have given the new department responsibility for all clinical skills teaching, including history taking, physical examination, differential diagnoses, and so forth. I did not want to hear further that primary care was not being done well enough here. We have got to have a vertically organized primary-care unit that is very strong, and very concentrated on teaching. Otherwise the students will become subspecialists. The second thing I tried and that failed was to organize clinical units horizontally. De facto they are now organized vertically. For example, in internal medicine, the endocrinologists and hematologists already have very little to do with each other and neither has anything to do with the gastroenterologists and abdominal surgeons. So I wanted to make one unit with 54 beds to include gastroenterologists, pediatric gastroenterologists, abdominal surgeons, certain types of radiologists and supportive pathologists, and a few others. I wanted to integrate house staff and make the unit financially self-supporting. I wanted to do the same thing for urology, neurosurgery, and electrophysiology and for hematology and oncology. A beginning was made but it has not been achieved as yet. In my opinion . . . although we must maintain departments . . . horizontal units must emerge for the purposes of patient care and medical student training.

McMaster's challenge since the mid-1980s has been to manage the ramifications inside—an accelerating faculty fee-for-service treadmill detrimental, as at UCSF, to student instruction—of increasingly strained relations outside, among Ontario doctors, patients, and government.

- People have all of a sudden got caught up in the fee-for-service treadmill at McMaster and there has been a huge shift in the socialization of physicians in these years. . . . It has been a terribly turbulent period in the relationship between doctors, patients, and the government. In a period of economic decline when steel mills and other factories are closing, there has not been much sympathy for physicians with six-digit incomes screaming across picket lines. The belief that doctors were healers and caregivers and do-gooders interested in people was harshly contradicted for the public by the contrasting image of physicians organized into crass labor unions. Another social change that has occurred in the last 5 years is that the public's awareness and understanding and questioning of basic epidemiological data has reached its highest level ever. These data and the differences among parts of the population that they reveal with respect to mortality and morbidity have led to a tremendous loss of faith in physicians. One of the ways that this has been reflected is that the Ontario government has recently decided to control health care spending by means of lowering fee schedules. Thus there is less and less sympathy with physicians as the public recognizes that these are not country doctors anymore but drivers of Mercedes. Within the medical school, this had the effect of changing the guard in the dean's office. We wanted a stabilizer, compromiser, someone committed to equity and fair distribution of limited resources. People saw [that] vice president Bienenstock was already doing the dean's job in other respects, including the academic.

Focused on adapting to a difficult environment, McMaster has paid less attention recently than it did in the early– to mid-1980s to MD program process and content, to rewriting problems, teaching the "burden of illness," incorporating epidemiological concerns. A "drift toward the residency" by clinical departments occurred as both cause and consequence of a marginalizing of MD program faculty, formerly the center of so much attention.

- [In the early 1980s there] was the organizational review of problems that made up the undergraduate curriculum. We did a close review of their content and structure and where they had failed. The curriculum truly was revised to reflect the "burden of illness" in our community. A core of us did the job.

• [I: How much has your department participated recently in the MD program?] Not much. We do have a problem in unit 3 in which an AIDS patient presents. He sees a so-called Dr. Bill in the north end of town. I was the model but did not know about the problem for 2 years and would not have formulated the problem in the way it was done! It was based on a fictitious case, after all. I myself would provide real cases. And some of the clinical stuff was out of date. [I: What does this indicate?] A bit of isolation, or maybe I should say not just a bit. There is no need to use fictitious patients. It is better to use real people and real experience. [I: Have you communicated that?] Yes. But there is strong competition in terms of resources. There are strong financial and clinical pressures, first of all, and second, the residency program in family medicine is the principal resource consumer in the department. Thus it is difficult to find faculty resources for the MD program. [I: Where does the department's primary loyalty currently lie?] At the residency program. It has drifted from the MD program to the residency program. The clinical demands on us have contributed to the drift toward the residency. It is a real push me–pull you, and the outcome always depends on who is pulling.

Notwithstanding nearly three decades' unswerving commitment to its signature innovation—small-group problem-based learning—the approach that made McMaster so original now lives less in the present and more in the past. One indicator that the old originality may be repossessed lies in recent consideration given by MD program faculty to incorporating traditional-curriculum content.

• The fundamental characteristic of the program, then as now, is problem-based learning in small groups. This, in a word, is still non-negotiable, even though some would like to loosen the grip of small groups and put everything up for grabs again. Still, the fundamental gospel has not changed at McMaster. The whole world is now following McMaster. The school began by challenging assumptions, but now we are the neo-orthodoxy and ironically we no longer have the ability to challenge our own assumptions. My own conclusion is that problem-based learning is a very expensive alternative that creates slightly better products. Nevertheless, learning is a highly individual process, regardless of the situations in which it occurs, and unless we admit this we will not be leading the next switch in the chain.

- We have broken down the parochial control of departments and integrated clinical material into the first years of medical education. In the recent accreditation of our second-year curriculum, what students ... valued most ... was the collegial atmosphere here and the high degree of interaction as well as diversity within the student body. They liked very much the contribution to their learning of their own peers. [I: What haven't you accomplished yet?] We have not yet integrated the good things from the traditional system. There were great strengths in the old system of teaching medicine. I am very concerned about the extent to which our students master the basic principles of our field, the molecular, biological, and genetic basic vocabularies. Historically, McMaster was founded by people who were fed up with the University of Toronto. Now we need to go beyond this "reaction" phase. We need to examine the 1960s as an era and as a philosophy. We cannot be grown-up flower children here. We must change. We risk being ossified otherwise. Incorporating change, we must also remember that our educational activity must be focused on the students in the program and on the best interests of the patient.

- In a pedagogical sense, the program probably still does address our original concerns, but without the same intensity and vigor as then. The spirit of the place has changed. This is undeniable. There is now less of the sense of collegiality, vitality, and excitement than there was. And another thing that I sense is that we have dogmatized the revolution, made problem-based learning and small groups almost the be-all and end-all of McMaster. We have experienced a sort of ossification. [I: Has this come about by external or internal causes primarily?] Internal factors primarily. We were looked up to because we were the experts, so our identity got tied up with this.

Sherbrooke's experiment geared up over the years that McMaster's experiment wound on in the fervent efforts of a coterie that designed in little over a year an utterly new student-centered, community-based, humanistic medical-education program modeled on earlier innovators but adapted to local needs.

- Out of the canvas group nominated by the dean and appointed by the vice dean in 1986, a program committee developed in 1987 to actually implement the program. The committee was led by Jacques Des Marchais and me. Our job was to understand the philosophy and method of student-centered, community-based humanistic medical education and to assure related faculty development. We set out to find responsible people for each unit and to start to translate ideas into practice. We organized a multidisciplinary group for each unit. There was one preclinical and 13 clinical units. In each group we got five to six people working. Soon the program committee was replaced by something called the validation committee, composed of six people nominated and appointed in the same fashion—one internist, one general medicine person, two basic scientists, that sort of thing—who went first to the meetings of the groups developing the big preclinical unit. We helped them learn how to write problem statements, for example. All the materials developed by the unit directors were sent to the validation committee for review, after which we discussed changes with the unit directors. These were mostly to cut and reduce content because we were now involved with problem-based learning, not just conventional teaching.
   [I: Were there any problems with the unit directors?] We were very diplomatic. We only offered suggestions, really. It was very collegial. But I may say that, for our credibility, we had a good deal of very valuable outside information, for example, from the University of Maastricht,

the University of New Mexico, McMaster University, and therefore a great deal of validity. Secondly, we got some money to run simulations involving three students who gave us 2 to 4 hours a week over the course of two summers, one after the first year of the program and the other after the second year. The students were unexperienced in problem-based learning and were experimental subjects with whom we tested the feasibility of the problems we were designing. We also invited the unit directors to observe the experimentation. The students gave us comments that were mostly about the appropriate level of the problem presented. They also reviewed the references that we assigned as part of the self-directed learning process. We use textbooks, and it is difficult to choose good textbooks. The students gauged the number of hours required for each assignment. The students were very generous in reviewing our materials and were proud to participate in the project, and we gained some credibility for this effort. In 1988 we realized that we needed a group to look at the more administrative aspects of implementing the program. This became known as the coordinating committee and was constituted by people in charge of the whole blocks, of which there were two and then three. At the beginning we were concerned just with daily problems, but in 1989 we started a review of each unit, beginning with the units that needed the most change, particularly the medical biology introduction and the clinical skills unit. Then, in 1989–1990 the vice dean nominated a fresh curriculum committee to work under him, charged to analyze the present with a view to the future. Their task was to redesign the new program, mostly on the basis of interviewing each unit head. At present, the coordinating committee meets 3 hours a month with the heads of each of the three phases, plus the clerkship director, plus the chair of the evaluation committee and someone from the administration. This committee still serves only to coordinate activity. The curriculum committee has become the future-oriented group and has a lot of influence on the coordinating committee, for example, in defining what self-directed learning means.

At Sherbrooke, as at UCSF, a new "research" dean soon found himself immersed in educational change. The sudden, nearly Cartesian implementation of the change at Sherbrooke gave many faculty, as it would at Hawaii, little time to adjust.

- Implementation came all at once, in September 1987. The former dean perceived it as the only way to succeed. [I: Why?] Because of the debate-debate-debate aspect. The dean thought that this would delay the change. He was a very clever man. The negative part is that it did not give people time to get used to the idea of an alternative education system as good or better than the existing one. It was first implemented in September of 1987, and I arrived in January 1988. Practically the day I arrived 50 people came one after another into my office to say, "Stop! We are only 3 months into the program. It still can be stopped." I did not come from a strong pedagogical background, but I did sense that the former dean made the right decision to change. Division directors asked me, only days after my arrival, what I thought of the new program. I said to them, "It will be a success and there is no way out." At that point I would say a third of the faculty was opposed, a third for, and a third neutral. [I: And the positive part?] It gave a clear message. It said that we are going to succeed and that we cannot go back.
- I was against implementing it all at once . . . for practical reasons. I had difficulty imagining that we could train all the teachers at the same time that we were developing the problems and everything else. I thought that we were being asked to believe in something that we had not seen and that we were being forced to take a direction from which there was no way back. I knew that all at once meant no going back. [I: Then did you favor a more experimental approach?] Yes, I did, but not like New Mexico, where it is 25 to 75% experimental-traditional. I wanted fifty-fifty experimental and traditional content for all students. I saw the basic sciences in a more traditional way and thought that these should constitute the traditional fifty percent of the curriculum. And I saw the clinical in the new way. I had the impression then that problem-based learning would be

better adapted to the clinical than to the basic sciences. I still believe that a lecture in the basic sciences is not a sin. [I: How was it then that the all-at-once people won?] They had the power and decision-making ability, though they did work very hard at consensus.

Certain clinical faculty and departments that had been peripheral in the old curriculum—family practice and general medicine in particular—were elevated and became central to the new curriculum as it was implemented.

- Many of those who first became involved had not been much involved with the old curriculum ... people, for example, in family practice, people who could not lecture before but in the new curriculum could teach general internal medicine very well. It was a group around the vice dean. With Jacques, there is never an official meeting. It is always in front of his office, always informal, always having coffee in flight. Well, I like it very much, but there are some who do not like it at all. Most decisions are made in brief, rapid contacts. Jacques does not want to talk about something for 3 hours. I once told Jacques that I was interested in bicycling and very shortly after I had an invitation to a 100–kilometer trip. It is the same with informal ideas concerning medical education and the new curriculum. It never takes 4 months to put something into practice. With Jacques, 3 weeks later, it is set up.
- The stock of family medicine in the faculty has certainly risen as a function of curricular change, while that of the basic scientists has fallen as a function of that change.
- To do this sort of problem-based, student-centered curriculum, you need a lot of staff. There are no lectures with one person handling 100 students. And, of course, our department also has postgraduate students. In 1987 it was clear that we did not have enough resources to do it. What saved me as department chair was my ability to recruit people, and to recruit particular types of people. It was, after all, the department of medicine that was most involved in the reform and which then grew the most. Since 1987 we have grown from 40 to 68 full-time faculty. The new curriculum

gave a role to people who had had no role before. Before the reform, we were considered the less academic people. With the reform, we have found a new way of being useful to the institution.

- In the traditional curriculum, the general internist was not really active in the preclinical years of medical education because all the subspecialists were there teaching things like the lung, the kidney, and so forth. The internists were very much involved in the clinical skills part of the undergraduate curriculum, however. Now with the new curriculum, the clinicians are very involved not only in clinical skills teaching but also in preclinical instruction, because as internists we can go from one unit to another in cardiovascular, neurology, gynecology, and so forth.

As at other schools where across-the-board changes were introduced, those basic scientists at Sherbrooke who felt that they might be sidelined by the changes constituted the greatest obstacle to implementing the changeover.

- Lack of basic science in the new curriculum has been a major concern. I share this point of view and I watched it very carefully. I had regular discussions with the program administrator and with the basic scientists. I also spoke with opponents of the program. I knew that the hardest thing would be to put the basic sciences into the program. I made sure I was there at meetings when there was a debate.
- The basic scientists are afraid of the undergraduate program in terms of its difficulty for them. It shocks them that you are asking them not to give lectures in what they know but to take an interdisciplinary viewpoint, which they have never faced or realized. In 1986–1987 I was surprised that, when you discussed integration and interdisciplinary points of view in thinking and conceptualizing with faculty, it came more naturally to the clinicians. The really thick walls came between the basic-science groups. They would work as neighbors but never as disciplines together. They never drink at the same pot of coffee. In meetings of a unit, they would fight among themselves, not about the subject but just because they liked fighting among them-

selves, because for them it is a way of life. It is how they get grants and space. So you have to fight their socialization if you want to involve them in interdisciplinary work. This has been decreasing, but it is still a problem.

- The more specialized, the more they do not like things now. So the basic scientists have more difficulty than the clinicians with the new curriculum. The basic scientists were the strongest opponents at first and they continued to fight it after it began. They included most of the bad tutors as evaluated by students in the first 3 years of the program. So for the basic scientists, the change was very difficult. To solve the problem we also put clinical scientists into teaching basic science.

But challenges also arose over physical space, converting teachers to tutors, and some residents' feeling that they were the ones now being neglected.

- We soon realized that curricular reform was one thing and physical structure another. Curricular reform means reorganizing physical space, and the physical limits soon became our biggest obstacle. This was solved, however. We took out all of the walls from the faculty building and reorganized offices. Now, instead of there being many little offices for professors, we also have meeting spaces to accommodate anywhere from 10 to a hundred people. Before, there was just no space for students. The other problem that we encountered was the training of professors. We had to retrain faculty to keep morale up. It was not that they did not know how to teach, rather that they had to learn how to tutor, how actually to motivate students. So retraining meant reviewing content and reviewing problems, Changing teaching method to problem-based learning meant switching people from a highly specialized—for example, in genetics—to an integrative point of view in teaching. Faculty now find their teaching more intellectually interesting. Teaching the same things for years becomes very boring, and so it is a stimulus to teach in new problem areas.
- The residents at Sherbrooke feel neglected. When the pro-

gram first began, everyone invested in pregraduate education. The residents felt old and that sort of thing. I am active in both pre- and postgraduate education, so I see it. It
is not that they are neglected so much as not seeing innovation at their level. Faculty are spending more time with
undergraduates, and you can really feel that here.

Adjustments of the new curriculum have included better
integrating the disciplines in basic-science instruction, maintaining supplementary lectures, even giving students a progress
exam, as at Mercer, Hawaii, and McMaster. Students are also
being offered more content in tutorials now.

- There was the "Maastricht problem." This is the question
  of content versus noncontent problems. What really
  changed us from the process viewpoint was the students.
  They want more content. Ironically then, self-directed
  learning is removing us from the strict method approach
  with which we started. My daughter, for example, is doing
  this curriculum here and she thinks that in the tutorials
  she is losing time. She says, "Let us have an open discussion and then go home and study instead of all this emphasis on method." It is just too rigid, she thinks; it is all feedback and group dynamics. She says that the clerkship for
  most students is a big relief.
- There have been a lot of minor adjustments at every level—
  there are many feedback loops built into every part of the
  program for both students and faculty—in areas such as tutor behavior, student evaluation, problem-writing, and content of problems. Earlier in the new program, the tutor was
  more passive and was more like an observer. There was an
  overreaction, I would say, to keep the tutor from beginning
  to lecture during a discussion. The role of the tutor has
  evolved since then and become more active, not in a way to
  give facts and answers but to challenge and to guide. It was
  beneficial at first to insist on extreme silence in the transition from the old methods, but now we are confident
  enough to return to a little intervention. We have [also]
  added some formative written exams in the middle of a session where there were none, for example, to increase the

question bank and give students a better sense of their progress. But there has been no change in the type of examination. Also, there has been some problem revision, saying, for example, that the specific problem is not well suited to what is needed. One or two of 10 problems have been modified or replaced in my areas, for example. Here too, the way the problems are delivered and the way students work them has remained exactly the same.

If the innovators at New Mexico benefited from having time and support to run the experiment and those at Mercer profited by starting from scratch and knowing their niche, the orchestrators at Sherbrooke succeeded by commanding an ample record of what had been accomplished elsewhere by the mid-1980s and by their methodic conversion–cooptation of faculty to a very new pedagogy.

- It was a very successful operation in the sense of planned steps. We had confidence in people to do it and they really did it. It is unbelievable what we accomplished. This is not to deny that there was a certain ambivalence in faculty commitment to the new program, a certain supportive attitude that goes up but then goes down, and this goes on even now.
- Leadership, organized leadership, the leadership provided by Des Marchais and Dumais, helped people progress toward their ideas. The role of Des Marchais was very important, especially that he came from the outside and had the personality to bring people together. In fact neither Dumais nor I could have succeeded in the way that Des Marchais did because we were insiders. One of the current risks that we have is that Des Marchais may still be felt as an outsider. If he had left in 1988 or 1989, there would definitely have been a backlash. As it is, by 1993–1994, there will be a small backlash. In effect then, three of us have implemented the program. Des Marchais brought in the ideas and the organization, I trained the teachers, and Dumais administered the program, the nuts and bolts implementation. We also had very clear ideas of what we wanted to attain in the end. This helped us very much. We were

not fuzzy as we started the canvas committee. We knew what problem-based learning was, and we knew what we meant by a community orientation. We may not have been sure of the details, but we had the major outline. Still, the basic-science people have always felt that they were left outside. We could have involved them more in the canvas committee. As I recall, there were only two or three basic scientists of 24 committee members. Maybe we should have given them more opportunity to voice their opposition and to respond to us.

- Our big worry was the participation of professors, but in fact this has gone quite well. Our other worry concerned whether students would bite the bullet and follow the new course of studies, and in fact they did. I worried a lot about whether all this would work, and I must say, yes, it has worked! In other words, there have been no big problems. I was surprised. The problems that we have had have all been surmountable. It was a lot of work, nights and weekends of work, but it all went rather well after the first adjustments. The only real difficulty was that it was a lot more work than we expected. We had to start from scratch to build all the problems that would guide the students.
- In small-group, student-centered learning, authority is largely transferred to the students and there are new rules of relationships among people. Students are involved in the process of evaluating not only themselves but also their tutors. In all, we now have much better communication, tutor to tutor, tutor to student, and tutor to administration, all the various permutations. It is a vast communicative process. Problem-based learning does do certain things intellectually. For example, students learn how to learn, not necessarily to learn content. But it is still difficult to convince faculty that facts are not the basic things to do in medical education. Citing the various psychological studies, they say that you need a large knowledge base to be able to reason properly about any specific matter. Thus, we are giving a mixed message to students and to faculty alike. Until now I would say, the decision has not been made by individual teachers to abandon content quite yet. There is still a hidden curriculum that resembles the old

curriculum. The new curriculum, I would say, is a success. But problems remain.

But the innovators at Sherbrooke were also aided by a historic and unusual dean-levered reward system that actually pays faculty to teach.

- The school opened in 1961 and graduated its first students in 1970. This was a period of expansion during which the school created specific programs, given that there was not enough money to hire in all the disciplines. And this is why the money is now put in one basket. The system was a means to make clear decisions among specific programs when you could not fund all of them during a period of expansion. The system was renewed for 10 years in 1979, and in 1989 it was renewed with no endpoint. The consensus is that it has worked for us very well. It is the key to how this institution has been able to change. At Sherbrooke, the method has been to reallocate the money in the basket and people know that, if a debate goes on too long, then the dean will call the shots. [I: So the system invites a benign dictatorship?] Exactly. If it is managed properly, then I take none of the decisions. In the system that we have, therefore, no one has ever gone to court. If the dean takes two wrong decisions in a row, at Sherbrooke he will not be there for the third. Then, at the end of the year, when the books are closed, the leftover always goes to the dean to distribute as a reward to those who have helped during the year. The dean can reward accomplishments, for example, in desired areas year by year, and these areas can be adjusted year by year. It is this managerial tool that is the key to my success. Without this tool, the new program here at Sherbrooke would not have succeeded after 5 years. There have been a number of things that I have tried to reinforce during this 5–year period. For example, I have rewarded faculty redevelopment efforts in this way, and very many faculty have gone back to school to learn new teaching tools. At other times, I have rewarded participation of faculty in tutorials. Faculty need to be motivated to participate in the new undergraduate curriculum, because it is often more fun for a physician to take care of the residents. But I have also rewarded research participation in this way. I have rewarded research productivity and I have rewarded departments in toto, not only individuals, according to their faculty redevelopment efforts, to their participation in tutorials, and to their research productivity. The system developed by necessity over the years in the process of hiring and developing subspecialties. The truth is that this funding mechanism can serve anything, including the present new curriculum.

- At Sherbrooke we have the big advantage of being able to reward faculty for teaching. In Montreal, for example, this would be much more difficult, because faculty are not paid for teaching. Here we did not have the problem of the reward system.

- We had a problem with money, with financing the new program. In a lecture system, there may be 100 students in one room receiving a lecture. Under the problem-based curriculum that same 100 students will be divided into 12 groups. Therefore, there is 12 times more teaching. This was not anticipated well. There had to be internal reallocations of the budget. [I: How was this done?] The financing system here is a peculiar one. It is entirely controlled by the dean. Every dollar is put into one basket and reallocated according to work done. Therefore we can and do actually pay people for what they do. It works so that if you do x you get $20,000 and if you do x, y, and z you get $100,000. This has been the key to changing the curriculum. For example, if the dean decides that there will be no more pay for lecturing, then lectures are no longer paid for. If the dean decides it is only tutorials that will be paid for, then people's income will derive from tutoring. When we were first implementing the new curriculum, I accepted 80% of the recommendations made by the department heads and the group practice plan people and, to 20% of them, I said no. [I: And what characterized the rejected ones?] Either they were not fair or they were not really needed.

At Sherbrooke, the threat of being closed in the early 1980s led to a fundamental innovation in medical education underwritten by a unique funding mechanism.

- In 1981–1982, the financial crisis hit Quebec and people were talking about a closing. The government did not actually acknowledge the possibility, but it was certainly in the air. There was talk of rationalizing the system, so that three schools might each enroll 130 students a year to produce 400 medical graduates, instead of four schools enrolling an average 100 students to produce the same number each year. When it was asked which of the four schools to close, it was always Sherbrooke that was the target. The impetus for our renewal thus came from the rumor situation. In 1982–1983, the dean went to Quebec City and asked, "What can we do to stay alive?" The Quebec prime minister was a former student of this school, Pierre Marc Johnson. This was a good coincidence for us. He said, "Make yourself essential, indispensable." This is how problem-based learning became the essence of Dean Pigeon's survival strategy. Then came the vice dean, Jacques Des Marchais. His was an extraordinary, not a regular, appointment. He came in at the senior level just to reform the medical-education program.
- In 1982 there was a decree that lowered all salaries of civil servants in Quebec, including university teachers. [I: Did this eliminate any positions?] No, not at the level of the medical faculty. There was termination of contracts, but this was at the university level. The medical faculty had 144 professor slots from the university, lowered that year by 13 but their occupants were not terminated at the medical school then because of a reshuffling we did with money from the hospital. This is when the medical practice plan came in here at Sherbrooke. This is when we started working with three pillars, first, about 130 posts from the university, then the new ones supported by clinical revenues, then those supported by external funding. This system allows the dean to shuffle from one to another and it works something like at the private universities. Thus we have a type of flexibility that would otherwise be blocked by the usual politics of fighting over slots and positions, which gets everybody involved, including the unions. So since 1982, the clinicians have had to sacrifice a lot of personal income. Since that year, we have had a system in place that

catches those who fall through the net. In effect, the norm is that you bring in your salary for 12 years, and after that the system has to pick you up if any problems develop. Thus, while a lot of our teaching positions come from the university, it was in the period after 1982 that other posts came in from various bursaries, including the government, the research council, private foundations, and the provincial medical research council. The system was put in place just in time, and it picked up a lot of the tab during the cutbacks at the university level. This is how we have stayed at between 170 and 180 faculty positions. As a matter of fact, we have recently increased to 200.

- First, the issue of survival has certainly been addressed. Now we are a leader in medical education. Second, the problem of teachers being bored. Now there are more enthusiasts and people who are proud to be here. [I: What proportion?] Seventy-five percent, I would say. Third, the problem of passivity of the students. They are much more active now. Whether they are more self-directed, I am not so sure, because the new program is quite organized and standardized. Nevertheless our students are much more involved in the program than they were before. Whether they are better problem-solvers, again I do not know. Some yes, some no, I suppose. Good students learn with any method. [I: And the average students?] I would say that in their learning abilities they are marginally better. Others say that the new program helps the best, does not hurt the average, and that the worst students stay the same. [I: So there has been no great transformation in students?] No, there has not been. But students now certainly do ask more questions. Do they read more? I am not so sure. They still want us to give them papers to read.

CHAPTER 7

Lessons

What have the innovators in the general professional education of physicians learned from their experience in the current reform cycle, and what do they have to teach the broader community of physician educators about the process of innovating?

Lessons relayed at Mercer are unmistakably related to the recently founded school's distinct mission as a private–public hybrid. If Mercer is the least mission-comprehensive of the 10 schools studied, then it is not surprising that the first lesson drawn concerns how challenging it is for a school obligated to train primary-care physicians for a state's underserved populations to keep graduates mission-consistent.

- The medical centers here in Macon and in Savannah ... have a range of residency programs, obviously. While they are supportive of our program, they are not totally congruent with our mission. They have interests both in supporting our mission and in being regional medical centers serving a population in the millions. This is how our students are exposed to highly specialized faculty. We have tried to stay on top of this. [I: How?] The chiefs of services at the medical center downtown and the chairs here of internal medicine and other departments are the same persons, for one thing. They all relate within these departments. They train our students and their own residents. Often the residents are being educated in specialties, orthopedics, for example. I do not have any problem with this as long as these residents are not my graduates. Furthermore, we will not sponsor fellowships in specialized internal medicine, though I am very happy with general internal medicine.

The hospital, of course, likes to see new specialists come to town. So while we will participate in the salary of core faculty fifty-fifty with the medical center, inasmuch as these are related to our medical-student education needs, we will not participate so in salaries of super-specialists of more value to the hospital's mission than to our own. At the most I will do 10% to their 90% for the salary of a critical-care person. [I: To stay on top of this situation, how much does this depend on face-to-face relations between you and leadership at the medical center?] Almost 100%, but leadership there is largely shared. Those who run the residencies are the same people or answer to the same people who answer to me for the medical education program.

Founded to be innovative in method as much as mission by innovators already steeped in problem-based, community-oriented physician instruction, Mercer teaches pedagogic pragmatism over purity in, among other areas, evaluating students.

• The McMaster thinking was that any quantitative evaluation should be only advisory. At Michigan State and Illinois, we had been through that already, and this is why we called the multidisciplinary examination diagnostic, not punitive. You have got to gather objective evidence and you have got to use it for the benefit of your students. At the same time, if you are not careful, the numbers become the dog, not the tail. Recently I would say that we have slipped into complacency. This is why we are now meeting to put more teeth into the oral exams and to train faculty accordingly. This is consistent with the 7– to 8–year review time that you need for faculty after a program gets started. Interestingly, at Michigan State they have just radically changed their curriculum once again, so nothing stays the same.

At Hawaii, it is the haste with which leadership sought to transform curriculum across the board that impresses faculty, basic science and clinical. Commandeered to change, Hawaii teaches how an administration may overreach, even with the best of intentions, its teaching faculty.

- There was very short lead time. I think that it was about 9 months from the time of approval to full implementation! We had a lot of loose ends, as you would expect. It was tough on the first class as well as on the faculty. For those not all that happy with recent and continuing changes, there is quite a bit of undercurrent discontent. The administration is fortunate here in that faculty is not very vocal. We have always had a strong dean here.
- It did go very quickly, there is no question about that. In terms of the complexity, I thought we were going too fast. But it is probably better that we did not give people time to mount all kinds of objections. There was a small group of people who said that change was happening too quickly. But it was in place by the time that they were ready to speak up. I did agree with the concept at the beginning that there was no way that we could do a double system, for example, with problem-based and traditional tracks. We thought that the McMaster system had proven that a strictly problem-based approach could succeed. [I: And that this way was adaptable here?] I thought that it was. My wife is in a public education and public health program. I had had first-hand experience of how it worked in a graduate program. I had also been chair of the curriculum committee for 4 to 5 years before problem-based learning. I was appointed by the dean. [I: And the change in turn was dean-driven?] Yes, compared to many. In fact this school would not have existed at all without strong deans.

    We introduced faculty to the tutorial system well and our tutor training was good at the beginning. But we did not follow up well. Follow-up consists in creating more interaction among tutors while they are tutoring. I would get tutors together regularly to deal with typical problems that come up in tutorials and how to deal with them. I would also say that the rewards system for teaching has got to be strengthened first. Being an outstanding teacher is still not the way to succeed here, and to young faculty-teaching is a necessary evil in order to survive. We should change this. [I:

How?] The problem in faculty promotion and tenure here is that there are department criteria, university criteria, but no medical-schoolwide criteria. But at neither the department nor the university level is teaching excellence well defined. The dean has appointed an ad hoc committee to get schoolwide criteria integrated into the university system. But I still do not understand quite how we implemented the program. It was a faith issue at first when we adopted the McMaster problems. Even so, we had to spend 4 months rewriting them to get them off the ground.

Utterly consistent with New Mexico's early-implemented, dean-engendered,ongoing primary-care curriculum experiment is the lesson, also drawn at Harvard, that a scientific community cannot in good faith deny a well-designed experiment, provided no already up-and-running programs or committed resources are too much diverted thereby.

- Well, I think that the important aspect in terms of change is to put forward to faculty that the new program is an experiment. Medical faculty have a background in doing experiments, so my way has been to say, "Let's run the experiment and get some results, then proceed on that basis to say yes or no." I tell faculty, "Look, there is just no starting with perfection, for an institution or an organization that wants to change." From an administrative point of view, you have got to get a consensus that it will be an interesting experiment to undertake, and that academics have a responsibility for education and not only for research. If you can get faculty to buy into the idea that everything is not going to be perfect from the start, or at any time for that matter, but that one can undertake responsible studies in education too, then you are on the way.

The challenge at New Mexico now, as it was at Harvard, is to generalize the experiment by joining the tracks, primary care and traditional.

- For [more conventional faculty] the pretheoretical assumption is that education equals transmission of information.

They think, "My value in education equals my expertise. I am just better able to organize this information." For them it is not the quality of the questions you ask, not the role of inquiry in the curriculum, but the organization and transmission of information. Thus they fear that they will have no place in a problem-based curriculum. The truth is, that we cannot do without these people even in the student-centered track, that we need them even more in a primary-care curriculum, because students regularly run up against the limits of their knowledge even more often than in the traditional curriculum. The problem with student-centered learning for these faculty is that they do not appreciate it unless they have seen it happen. Most of us who have seen it happen live for the time that we tutor again. I actually get very down between sessions.

Minnesota is the big public medical school inside a major, highly differentiated, research-oriented academic health center that teaches how difficult it is to integrate biomedical and clinical science instruction in a balkanized, departmental environment.

- While I have been coordinating the basic sciences, we have gone through several course directors. [Not every department head] is like the new head of pharmacology [who] holds the view that it is better to integrate and coordinate than to ask simply, "How many hours do we get?" [I: Who does not want this sort of integration of basic science and clinical to happen?] I do not know anybody in a position of power who does not want it. Some typically older faculty who may have been successful for 20 to 30 years and do not want to change anything may not want this. You know, you have been teaching something for a long time and you have a very strong feeling that it must be taught and must be taught your way! You think that students just cannot practice without what you have done all these years! [I: So it is generational?] Yes. Or a person who has a lab, says I teach head and neck, what else am I going to do? There are these failures to adapt, too, whatever the age. But then when you start talking to them about the options and sometime later you hear a knock on the door and someone comes in and says, "I thought about it. Let's try this or that." So people do come around.

Case Western Reserve, an innovator since the Eisenhower era, has a perspective to impart that no other medical school can match. Fortunately, there are faculty still active who may bring that perspective to bear, by warning how deeply subverting discipline-departmentalism can be to general professional medical education.

• [I: Could any lessons be brought from the 1950s and 1960s into the 1990s to inform current innovation process?] First, it is important that department chairs pick people and leave the educational programs up to them rather than try to run the whole thing themselves. Nowadays the department chairs have budgets bigger than the whole school budget was here in 1952. This means that you must be a good picker. Second, the idea that education be separate from department structure was a very good thing. This became very clear to me when I was chair of the committee on medical education. Third, have the curriculum coordinators rotate and thus keep the foment going. This also allows coordinators to serve and then return to their departments. Fourth, listen to the students! Just listen to them. But this is all very difficult to assure, because the department chairs are reluctant to allow their people into the educational establishment because they fear that it will damage careers or that they will be lost to the department. The chairs are outraged when good people get involved in education. So here we are at a time when a new national system of medical care will be devised in the next 4 years, yet no one in the medical school or in the teaching hospitals is discussing how to change accordingly. Even at Huff Norwood Hospital, all I hear is, "We are not going to be the guinea pigs in community-care medicine." The problem is to get a forum inside the medical school to discuss new health care delivery systems. We are hardly tapping this, and so the primary model of ambulatory-care medicine is still the outpatient clinic, which is a very clumsy way of delivering care.

Dartmouth's innovation to date has put a quarter of all clerkships into outpatient settings. In this, one administrator learned the importance of enlisting students and taking the time needed to manage control-minded department chairs.

- I learned that you have to look carefully at who needs to be involved in the collaboration. The key first of all was to involve the students. If the students had been excluded and then said, "Oh no," then the chairs could have said "Oh no" more easily. Second, time was important. There had to be time enough to work out the knots. It took 3 years to iron these out and talk it through. Since then we have spent a lot of time in meetings, clerkship meetings, discussing horizontal issues, issues that bear on all the clerkships, for example, why communication skills were only part of the psychiatry clerkship. We have put a lot of horizontal or common content into all the clerkships, for example, in patient-teaching skills. We videotaped students trying to teach a simulated patient something about health care. They are evaluated three times during the clerkship. Besides these two elements, collaboration and horizontal content, a third will also be important to our clerkship effort, namely, the integrated curriculum that we are currently discussing in the new directions committee. Now everyone is thrilled that we are known as a leader in outpatient clerkship medical education. The dean is very impressed, and the AAMC has recently asked him to be on an outpatient committee. In the new directions committee we are throwing around a lot of outpatient stuff. We recognize that we will have to go out into the community. I am pushing for a first-year clerkship experience with community practice physicians, not with our super-studs at the hospital. My question is, can I find that many doctors for 84 to 90 freshman medical students, especially when these community physicians have always been shunned by the ivory tower?

Dartmouth also teaches that money, foundation support, for example, may be no less a prerequisite to innovation capacity for smaller, lesser-endowed medical schools.

- Not until big money comes in will we go to real educational change here. My hope is that with private donors or the new Koop Institute this will bring in enough to make our ideas implementable.

Harvard learned that putting parts of its experimental track into general use by the early 1990s was costly, first, in diluting commitment to problem-based learning, and second, in institutionalizing the new role of full-time teacher.

- First, it involved moving away to some extent from the commitment to problem-based learning. [I: Why?] Because many faculty were not convinced that it is an appropriate way to learn the sciences related to medicine. That is why I like the book *Mathematics Insight and Meaning* by Jan de Lange Jzn, which shows that problem-based learning works in math! I now tell my faculty that, if it works in the most rigorous of the sciences, then problem-based learning can also work in the natural sciences. Second, and even more of a cost from my perspective, is the extent to which it impeded the development of faculty teams made up of people who considered their job in medical education to be conceiving and implementing the whole rather than some specific part of the curriculum.

Department organization hinders thinking about the educational whole in contrast to the subdisciplinary parts at Harvard no less than at Minnesota and Case Western Reserve.

- I think of medical education in two ways. First, I think of it conceptually in terms of content, all that we think any physician should know, and in terms of process, how best to develop that knowledge. Conceptualizing what a physician should know and how best to develop that knowledge really requires unending attention by a responsible faculty. Second, I think of medical education organizationally. By this

I mean, how can a faculty best organize to get the job done? Thus in 1920 it may have been appropriate to have the department structure do it, when there was one full professor in each department and these 20 or so could get together, know each other, and talk it over around one table. But in 1990 the department of medicine alone at the Brigham and Women's Hospital very often has over 300 faculty! And it is now the case that nephrologists do not talk to cardiologists and cardiologists do not talk to endocrinologists. Now even ophthalmologists have subspecialized, specialists in the cornea, anterior chamber, lens, retina, and so forth. No one is thinking about the whole. And it is the same in the basic sciences.

Indeed Harvard's concept of the medical-education society seems inspired by a critique of departmentalism very close to that, described above, which underlay Case Western Reserve University's effort in the 1950s and 1960s to separate education from department structure.

- The idea of a society is to create a cadre of faculty drawn from the disciplines and specialties but who think not just in disciplinary terms but also interact in building up a general view of medicine in the most inclusive sense.

University of California, San Francisco (UCSF), most like Harvard, but also like Sherbrooke, teaches how critical leadership is—school- and department-level—to general professional medical education innovation within a big many-sided academic medical center in which the common medical student might otherwise be overlooked.

- First, and absolutely necessarily, is strong support for change from the top. Unless the dean and the department chairs want to change, there will be no change. I was there at Harvard when [Tosteson] got the religion on that committee. The fact is that every department has students in whom it is more interested than medical students. For the basic scientists, these are the PhD candidates, and for the clinicians this is the house staff. The school is judged nationally on how well these do. Medical students do not have any natural constituency. They are the transient recipients of the attention of faculty in contrast to PhDs and house staff. Therefore it requires a strong dean and a strong central focus to bring about curriculum change. This is a little ironic if you consider that the real reason for medical schools is to pay attention to medical students. But it is also true. Without that central drive, it is easier to pay attention to the natural constituents.

Experience at UCSF, in efforts to implement problem-based learning, shows how difficult it is to innovate in the clinical phase of a less-integrated, traditional medical curriculum. It likewise underscores how students' mind-set at a ranking medical school may present as great an obstacle as faculty's to changing biomedical science instruction.

- I think there were several major mistakes. First, we just assumed that clinical education could be problem based. As a result, we have too many balls in the air now and are trying to cover each with grants. It is very difficult to get clinical departments to change their educational process, much more trouble than we thought. We should have dealt with this from the start. Second, we assumed that the behavioral sciences could just be integrated into problem-based learning. This was not the case, in fact. Students still come in with the standard premedical mind-set. So we had to make a separate behavioral-science unit. We were wrong to think that students did not even need a psychiatric clerkship. Third, we assumed that students would just pick up on this learning method. We had little problem with faculty learning, but the students wanted to traditionalize the tutors. They wanted to please the faculty. So we had to create student training workshops. So there had been some surprises.

The high regard, indicated by widespread emulation, in which McMaster is held around the world, does not copy so well at home, isolated as the MD program was over the course of the 1980s within a big health sciences faculty. A messianic program that for so long sent such talented paradigm-shifters out into the medical-education community, now recognizes how little attention it was paying to its home base over just the period when the revenue imperative, as at Case Western Reserve, surpassed the teaching mission.

- I think that the major message is that we have not yet spent enough time, effort, and money on putting together basic infrastructure for the MD program. A very apt analogy would be the military one, where there are 10 troops keeping every one soldier fighting. It is this sort of supportive infrastructure that we need to keep the MD program working, to keep it student centered and community based. What we have not got right yet is the leadership role. The MD program chair to date does not have the right funding and needs a secure financial base. Then, too, the MD chair must likewise be put on a sound footing. Her funding is like a dog's breakfast, 10% from here, 5% from there, and so forth. The lesson is therefore that critical positions like the MD chair must not be funded by dog's-breakfast means, and that there must be the resources for much, much more faculty development activity.
- The thing that has changed, compared to the original McMaster spirit, is the horizontal dimension of the program, the teaching dimension, for example. Before 1976, this place just vibrated. Then the faculty practice plan dealt a major blow. In 1987, I gave a seminar at the Ben Gurion Medical School. I was doing some research there for my book, and I said to these folks, "Look at all the horizontal stuff at McMaster. Look at all the informal networks, the kind of networks that run from the synagogue to the doughnut shop," I joked. I asked them what they thought was special about McMaster, and they all said problem-based learning, the community orientation, that sort of thing. I said, "Okay, but look at all the horizontal functions, look at what the program does informally." Then I said, "And now look at how much the practice plan did-in these functions." A nice old man, Aaron Antanovsky, sat in the back corner of the room. He was involved in the late 1940s and 1950s in the kibbutz movement. He said, "You

know, this all reminds me of the kibbutz. At first we were young and idealistic and poor. But we were also strong and interactive. Then we became bigger and older and wealthier and less strong and less interactive." [I: What advice would you give to other programs that were considering changes of the sort that McMaster represents?] First of all, you must have stable leadership, and leaders must be strong people who are widely trusted. Second, do not get too big, because you have got to share certain values. Third, you must constantly reinvest in the program. Fourth, you must not take for granted the participation of people working in the system. People cannot think they are being taken for granted.

The change at Sherbrooke teaches that if knowledge is power, compromise on all but principle is good practice. For the complete change that Sherbrooke and Hawaii represent, dean and core-group commitment is essential, but at Sherbrooke there was also a real threat to survival and related consensus for change as well as the timely arrival of an outsider.

- First, be ready to compromise on many things, but never on principle. Second, be sure of the dean's commitment. The dean has to be behind the design. Third, develop good relations within the core of reform people. Interact at work, but also socially and personally. Bertrand Dumais and I ended up sleeping in the same room together over the course of this process many times, at AAMC meetings, here overnight, at the medical faculty, and other places. We really were part of a team. Thus, you need to be able to count on very committed people, people willing to take risks, people who have something else to do if it does not work out. Finally, be confident about the outcomes, know the literature, know the experiences of other places with problem-based learning. It is this knowledge that is the origin of your confidence.
- First, do not try to make change if nobody has change in mind. Talk about real educational change must be in the air among the teachers. Otherwise you have a very dry ground. Second, get the dean's commitment and organize

leadership. This is very important. Start with the convinced, but always try to widen the group. Third, consider bringing in an outside prophet, but one likewise supported by insiders. Here, Dumais was a well-respected insider who was fully supportive of the outsider Des Marchais. Finally, do not try to change a medical school only with the advice of PhDs and specialists in education. All of us here, the core of those who brought the new curriculum, were physicians working in medicine. Thus, MDs who are also interested in education should be at the center of the process.

Sherbrooke innovators coopted fence-sitters into designing, then implementing, change even as they took care that such activity not be seen to supplant other vital functions like research. They painstakingly maintained clear lines of real authority and accountability and arranged to reward desired new behaviors during implementation. In retrospect they conclude that with determined leadership, a real and recognized need to change, and willing faculty participation, anything can be accomplished. With Maastricht, Sherbrooke made big change the virtue in necessity.

- First, get people convinced of the benefits of such a change and have them participate in the process. Second, get the manpower to support the entire implementation with no negative impact on other activities, such as research and professional involvement.
- First . . . if there are not clear lines of governance, if people are not directly accountable to someone, then do not do it. Here there were clear lines of authority and accountability, and clear lines of reward. This is necessary to accomplish a big reform. With this in place, you can do anything. Second, you must have the human resources. You must have the desire to reform the curriculum. At the present time, in the English universities in Canada, for example, McGill, they do not really see any reason to reform. Likewise, at the University of Montreal, staff do not feel the need. They look at it only as reform for the sake of reform. Here it was reform with a real reason. We were searching for an identity, and there was also the issue of survival. What I am

saying is that you have to have a strong reason. I think that the University of Maastricht was also in a search for identity. They were the small guy in contrast to the big guy in Amsterdam. Problem-based learning gave them a place and a way to become a big guy themselves. Third, you need to find a big boy scout. For 7 years at Sherbrooke, starting in the late 1970s, nobody would do it, nobody would be the leader. Then we found Jacques Des Marchais. He was looking for a lab for his ideas. We gave him the opportunity, and he gave us the reform. It was a very good bargain. [I: Was the change more a matter of survival or identity by then?] By the time Jacques came it was more an identity than a survival issue, even though the fear certainly was present. Now we do not fear anymore, because we are good for at least another 25 years. The motivation to change, I would say, is never for good, rational reasons. At the University of Montreal he had tried to implement his ideas but without success. The first thing he told me when he came to Sherbrooke was, "You have everything to do it here." To us, it was not obvious, but to Jacques it was.

P~ART~ 3

Innovation Subjects

Finally, how do the students, the subjects of these efforts, evaluate their schools' curriculum experiments? In chapter 8, we will answer the question by listening closely to their characterizations, first, of what was most, and what was least, beneficial in their instruction to date; and, second, what they imagine, several years into practice, will then appear to have been most and least beneficial.[1]

Common themes emerge at all schools in what students consider most beneficial in their MD programs. This is our first key finding. Invariably, they like those parts that encourage individuation, professional and personal, on the one hand,[2] and connection, to students, faculty, patients, and communities, on the other.[3] The diversity of student bodies, in the several ways in which these may be diverse, is also prized wherever it is found.

Common themes also emerge in what students consider least beneficial about their MD programs, but in this, our second finding, two sets of schools are identifiable. The first set includes the smaller, mission-distinct schools where more wholesale innovation has been undertaken. Mercer, Hawaii, New Mexico, McMaster, and Sherbrooke have variously developed the new pedagogical options that appeared in the 1970s and 1980s—small-group, problem-based, student-centered, basic- and clinical-science-integrated, patient- and community-oriented medical instruction—and innovated profoundly in medical education. With differences of emphasis, probably due to the suddenness of the change process, students at these schools dislike those parts of their programs that provide too much new pedagogy[4] and too little standard instruction.[5]

The second set of schools includes the larger, mission-comprehensive schools where more bounded innovation has been chosen. Thus Minnesota, Case Western Reserve, UCSF, and, though smaller,

Dartmouth have selected more narrowly from among the same new options, at the same time preserving, in part or whole, rather conventional lecture-lab-clinic curricula. Even Harvard's broad-scope New Pathway cannot help being mitigated by the advanced biomedical research and practice environment in which it is located. Students at these schools dislike those parts of their own programs that provide too much standard instruction[6] and too little new pedagogy.[7]

Those who would change the conventional curriculum, especially at larger mission-comprehensive medical schools, the majority in North America, should heed our first finding. Students invariably appreciate even limited efforts, wherever these are made, to effect small-group problem-based independent learning, curriculum integration, and early exposure to patients. This is so much the case that where these efforts are least in evidence, students are most anomic. In this, the limiting case is certainly Dartmouth, newest at innovation of the ten cases studied here. But students' resounding acclaim at Minnesota for the one instance, in an otherwise standard instruction, of integrating biomedical and clinical science instruction is also indicative. Conversely, where efforts of these sorts are most in evidence, at Harvard and McMaster for example, students are least anomic, most attached to and identified with the institution's innovation.

Those who would make more sweeping changeovers of curriculum might in turn heed our second finding. At the more wholesale innovator schools studied here, students, who must nevertheless compete for residencies in the unreconstructed postdoctoral world, want effective instruction in any case, whether it comes from a tutorial, a lecture, or a lab. In this, the limiting case is certainly Hawaii, where the abruptness of change left too many discrepancies between the new and the old pedagogies. The variably comparable objections raised by students in problem-based curricula at Mercer, New Mexico, Harvard, McMaster, and Sherbrooke are also revealing.

NOTES

1. For context, each respondent is identified at the end of each passage by curriculum year (U.S. 1–4, Canada 1–3), race or ethnicity (*w*hite, *b*lack, *a*sian, *h*ispanic, *n*ative american), sex (*f*emale, *m*ale), and age. The identification (2wf24) thus indicates a second-year, white, female, 24-year-old student.

In commentary to text in chapter 8, "they" means "one or several students" questioned.

2. As in controlling one's own schedule, not wasting time on lectures at Mercer; self-directed learning expected and emphasis on learning process at Hawaii; learning how to learn, or just the chance to learn medicine, even in one's 30s, at Minnesota; independent learning and curricular flexibility at Case Western Reserve; hard-won individual competence and off-campus opportunities at Dartmouth; the personal and intellectual independence and method training in medical reasoning at Harvard; the curricular flexibility, encouragement of self-identification, joint degrees, and fifth years at UCSF; being admitted without a strictly premedical preparation, getting respect from faculty, choosing electives at McMaster; self-directed learning, free time, freedom of scheduling, appreciation of individual differences at Sherbrooke.

3. As in cooperating, not competing, in tutorial, small-group instruction even in clinics, and acquiring patient communication skills at Mercer; psychosocial and clinical orientation and accessibility of faculty at Hawaii; faculty commitment to teaching, whole-person and prevention orientation, camaraderie, cooperation at New Mexico; early access to patients and clinical correlations at Minnesota; faculty dedication, student cooperation, and early patient exposure at Case Western Reserve; exceptional courses at Dartmouth; orientation to patients, mutual support and sharing among students, and the ambience in tutorials at Harvard; the learning environment, pass–fail option, student interaction and cooperation at UCSF; small-group problem-based learning, the integrated curriculum, common-belief system at McMaster; integration of learning into hospital life, participatory approach to learning, integration of science and real problems, and the humanistic approach at Sherbrooke.

4. As in ruling out lectures, discouraging competition at Mercer; being guinea-pigs for new curriculum at Hawaii; learning too much forest and not enough trees in the primary-care curriculum at New Mexico; tutorials that break down, the cumbersome process of students evaluating tutors, and immersion in education jargon at McMaster; unevenness in quality of tutors and not knowing quite what is expected at Sherbrooke.

5. As in too little lab science and procedural medicine instruction at Mercer; too little chance at competitive residencies due to being labeled at Mercer and New Mexico; too few basic-science details at Hawaii; not enough conventional teaching at McMaster; too little basic-science detail, too little formal educational structure and related uncertainty at Sherbrooke.

6. As in fragmentary science lectures with little patient perspective, inattentive clinical instructors, a divisive honors system at Minnesota; curricular rigidity at Case Western Reserve; too many lectures, too little mentoring, too much impersonality, hazing, test-taking, and grading at Dartmouth; the pace and antiseptic, nonmedical tenor of basic-science lectures at Harvard; too much overwrought, achievement orientation at UCSF and Harvard.

7. As in the lack of legal-economic content in clinical instruction at

Minnesota; too little community medicine, epidemiology, doctor–patient instruction at Dartmouth; the pedagogical noncorrespondence between New Pathway and clinical instruction and the uneven quality and commitment of tutors at Harvard; too traditional, high-tech clinical instruction after the first biennium at UCSF.

CHAPTER 8

Student Evaluations

Mercer nurtures its all-Georgian students, who most appreciate controlling their own schedules, not wasting time in traditional classes, cooperating rather than competing in tutorial-based learning, and being instructed in small groups even in hospital clinical rotations. Mercer attends closely to students who will soon serve in far reaches.

- It is the free time that I have here, compared to a traditional program, that has been most positive for me. My friends at the Medical College of Georgia waste a lot of time in class but still have the same study as I have. (2wm27) I like the tutorial program very much, the personal aspect of it, the smallness of it, the relations with professors and students. I can go to a professor at any time. It is these personal things that are of benefit to my learning. Everybody helps each other here. There is not an attitude of competitiveness. I have friends at the Medical College of Georgia who do not know any of their classmates. (2wf24) I went to Emory [University] as an undergraduate. I always had large classes. My personality is, I do not speak unless spoken to. The small-group tutorial here has forced me to get to know people. Otherwise I might not have. I think that students pulling for each other varies from class to class. The second-year class is exceptional in this. (3wf25) I especially agree about the small groups and access to faculty. I have also found there are opportunities at the hospital in clinical rotations for small-group work. I am in surgery. At other schools the clerks and even the residents basically just hold the retractors. Here it depends on how much you want to do.

At the Medical Center downtown, there is less scut work, busy work, more real work. (3wm27)

The family theme emerges, too, in how students imagine Mercer will seem to have benefited them as practitioners, 6 to 8 years hence.

- Eight years from now I imagine that I will be in Cordele, Georgia, as a pediatrician. I have been talking with the town. The option is a group or private practice there. I imagine that, being there, the most positive thing about my time here will have been my colleagues, especially in general surgery. I have made very good friends here, especially among residents who have affected me more than Mercer faculty with respect to what I will practice. (3wf25) I have no idea where I will be except that I will be in Georgia. I will likely be in a smaller town than Macon, for example, Statesboro, which has about 30,000 population. [I: In primary care?] Yes, probably family practice and some medical oncology. I am not a terribly inward person, but I do feel that by this experience I have learned to relate well to patients. It has taught me that right underneath the medical skills is your relationship with the patient. (2wf24) I will be in a town of say 25,000 to 30,000 within 30 to 40 minutes' ride of a major metropolitan area. I will be doing something in internal medicine or going into endocrinology or cardiology. [I: What will have worked for you at Mercer?] Having had a lot of free time to pursue my own interests and having had some great friends. I never thought that I would have this much fun in medical school. I have been to a Mardi Gras and to the World Series. I have been in a good class that gets along very well. (2wm27) I will be practicing somewhere in Southeast Georgia, in a small town of 15,000 or less. I will also be mission-compliant. I will probably go into family practice or internal medicine bordering on general practice. For me, it will have been the closeness with people. These are some of the best friends I have ever had . . . it is almost like family. Here you have to get along, work together. It is a lot of work, but you also have time here not to study. Also, our training in the sec-

ond 2 years here will make the residency easier than it will
be for traditional graduates. The residents I meet say how
elsewhere the clerks do mostly scut work. (3wm27)

But students object that the program lacks lab work, possibly to discourage specialization, offers too little practical and
procedural medicine at first, unnecessarily rules out lectures,
and discourages competition. Tutors are careless of students,
and clinic patients protest that they are given second-class
treatment. Landing competitive residencies may be difficult
coming out of such a little-known school, they worry, and acquired debt too great for the lesser-paying primary-care practices that they will enter. There is the hint here that Mercer
will be challenged to keep students mission-compliant.

- Anatomy laboratory is not required. You have the opportunity for this but it is not required. Likewise in histology, we
  do have labs at our disposal, but a lab should be required
  for both histology and anatomy. Visualizing these materials is very important. I think that the reason that labs are
  not required is because the faculty thinks that none of us is
  supposed to be a specialized surgeon anyway. (2wf24) You
  can graduate from this school without taking blood, or
  starting an IV. This is really scary ... more scary to me
  personally because I tend to isolate. (3wf25) First, I carry a
  much heavier debt load than I would have at the Medical
  College of Georgia. And they are now limiting us to primary care when we come in. Second, for those who want
  competitive residencies, Mercer is less well-known than
  Emory, not to mention Johns Hopkins or Harvard. Third,
  sometimes you feel that you are there in a clerkship to be
  slave labor, especially in surgery. At Mercer you see patients and that is it. You do not see patients at other
  schools because the residents and fellows come first. At
  Mercer, you see them right away and the responsibility is
  yours. (3wm27) This is especially evident in the medical
  center clinic because the population is indigent. I have often heard people say, "Why are you doing all this? This is
  the clinic." I was taking blood pressure at the time and it
  really mattered. (3wf25) The same thing happened to me. I

was chastised for doing such an extensive workup for a clinic patient. (3wm27)

- Mercer encourages students to do mediocre in the first 2 years by not wanting to advocate competition. Then there are the little things. There are some professors who cannot ever assign correctly. And there are others whose study guides are full of errors and mispagination. [I: What do you attribute this to?] They do not investigate or research new volumes. They are too focused on research. They are not up to date and they miss things. But my major complaint is that the school advocates no lectures and cancels things like optional training of this sort in pathology at the same time that, in the community science program, there is a very boring lecturer who goes on and on with a lot of community junk. It is a real waste of time. (2wm26) [I: So you all have no problem with lectures when they are efficient?] No, no problem. [All] like lectures in the pathology optional training. Sometimes lectures are very efficient. (2wm26)

Still, when Mercer students imagine what will appear, several years into practice, to have least benefited them in their medical education, the positive prevails.

- I honestly cannot think of anything consequential that I will not remember fondly. (3wf25) I do not see anything negative of importance for the future. (2wf24) The biggest thing is all the loans. With two degrees, in pharmacy and medicine, both from private schools, I will have a large debt. (2wm27) I do not see anything really. (3wm27)

Hawaii shocks, then exhilarates, its largely Asian students. They come to value self-directed process-oriented learning, the orientation to psychosocial and clinical medicine, and the accessibility of faculty. Inhibited at first by the value placed on group harmony in Asian culture, most get the hang of small-group problem-based learning. Hawaii wants students self-actuating in time for generalist practices in urban and rural island communities.

- Faculty are eager to be resources and really seem to be concerned. (2af30) [I: What would you say to a prospective student who likes the idea of studying medicine in Hawaii?] I would ask how self-motivated they are, how able to work alone. The group only meets twice a week and thus there is a lot of studying alone. (4am28) I would ask whether they care about getting to the destination or whether it is the journey itself that they are interested in. When the school accepts people who are not process-oriented, it really hurts the group's practice. It frustrates everyone. (3wm36) The school is not good for people without a psychosocial orientation. (2af30) I would tell them that a good science background helps, but that I also had a friend with a religion and music major who just matched in neurology at his first choice. (2am26)
- Problem-based learning was a big shock to me, at first, but it turned out pretty nice. I felt the first day we did tutorial that not even the tutor knew how to approach the problem. One person in the group actually physically turned away because he did not know what role to play. It took about 3 weeks to get the group going. You tend to sit back, not risking stepping on other people's toes. You have to get to know the members, see how each might end up. Sometimes it never gels. Once I remember there were two very vocal people with opposing points of view and three quiet people. In that case the tutor did not help because he was equally vocal. (4am28) Culturally and socially it was a difficult process for me getting started. For Asians it is a value not to let anyone lose face. (2af30) Yes, harmony is often more important. We have had problems when it comes to relaying important information and critiquing. Sometimes not only the students but also the tutors do not know how to do it. For this reason, the formal review after 12 weeks can come as a shock. (4am28) We work here on a trimester system, three semesters of 12 weeks each. At the end of each trimester, there is evaluation of individuals and of programs. (2am26)
- In your first year you can go up to the chair of the department of pediatrics and ask a question and get help. I do not know how many places you could do this. It is really like

being in a candy store, considering the list of people you can use as resources. The sky is the limit. You can go into labs and ask the directors what they are doing and they will show interest in your question. (4am28) [I: So if I like learning on my own, and I am willing to approach faculty, a nonscience background is not a problem?] Yes, but do not assume that you have covered all the bases here for licensure. (3wm36) [I: So problem-based learning is independent learning but you still have to pass the boards?] Yes, and there is a lag between our type of program and board content. We are ahead of the boards . . . though they are gradually coming to have more clinical content now. (2am26) There is 9 weeks' elective time to prepare for the boards and over this period faculty do give very helpful colloquia. (2af30) We had the impression that the school would provide us something structured to help us prepare, but they said, "You organize it, you prepare it." We were angry but we did find two students to organize everything and we got through the boards. It is not so much the pedagogy per se that the school is concerned with, for example, tutorials versus colloquia. Rather it is whether it is student driven or not. If it is not student driven, the faculty are not likely to go along. (4am28) In my class . . . those with an internal locus of control tend to unfold into whatever they are doing. In this regard I think that the part of unit 2 on how to read the scientific literature critically, and the part of unit 5 where there is a week of 2–hour sessions on critical appraisal, are very helpful. (3wm36)

Empowerment in having learned self-direction is what students imagine they will most appreciate about Hawaii in retrospect once they are practicing physicians.

- Most valuable will be that there is nothing in medicine that I cannot make my own if I devote time to it. This is the view that I am acquiring here. (3wm36) It will have been my ability to work with peers, even if I do not like them much, and that I am not afraid to approach doctors with what I do not know. (2am26) I will have gained and broadened my perspective as much as acquired the tools to do medicine. Perspective is what problem-based learning emphasizes, the holistic view of people. I will value the fact that I have acquired a way to learn, as much as a whole lot of details. (2af30) Most positive will be empowerment. In our class we had to fight for it. It was almost a one-way deal. There was so much resistance by the administration. But a good tutor, for example, mine in the life-cycle tutorial, can really play an important role in your education in this regard. In this way I stopped thinking just doctor–doctor and started thinking person–person. (4am28)

Even so, there is anger among students who were experimental subjects for the hastily implemented new curriculum at Hawaii, as well as discontent with related discrepancies, such as between program goals and admissions policy. They resent lingering faculty confusion concerning whether to evaluate students individually or collectively and dislike the third-year honors program, considered a holdover from the old system. Curriculum so quickly and completely altered is prone to such inconsistencies.

- The first class to do problem-based learning pioneered for subsequent classes. They did not even have a library, a computer room, a laser printer, anything, and there were big holes in the curriculum, for example in embryology. (3wm36) A lot of people in our class . . . were very angry about what we had to go through. (4am28) In my view, the admissions committee has not caught up with the program. In this type of program, personality is an issue too. For this program, you have got to be interested in becoming a better person as much as a better doctor. (2af30) Your peers help mold you here. I am constantly affected by people in this class. (4am28) For me the biggest shortcoming is the lack of solidarity on the part of faculty over test and measurement issues, for example, over how [we] will be assessed. Faculty need to quit bickering and get it together concerning the end-of-the-year performance test. (3wm36) Yes. At the end of unit 2, things fell apart when they moved to a 25% multiple choice and 75% essay format. (4am28) [I: How do these evaluations affect the cooperative spirit here?] We were told that we would be graded individually in unit 4 in contrast to being evaluated on how the class did. And this made people stingier in helping other people in their studies. (2af30) This was not good. It only fostered competition. (2am26) Yes, and it is in the second year, just when people are preparing for the boards, which brings a lot of schism into the class anyway. (2af30) But it is pass-fail, you must admit. (4am28) I am in the third year and there is an honors part of the clinical rotation. That really starts the competition. Evaluations go almost word for word into your dean's letter. So people vie for cases. Honors is a holdover from the traditional program here. (3wm36)

Learned cultural inhibitions and guinea-pig status recur in what students imagine they will least appreciate about Hawaii in retrospect. One thinks that the details will appear to have been glossed over in biochemistry and pharmacology.

• Least valuable [will be] that in these years I will have lost my ability to be candid . . . because of how much negative emotion and candor is repressed in this culture. It is so much a part of Asian culture. The spontaneity that I once had will be gone because of these 4 years. It is a cultural fact of this program. (3wm36) For me, it will be the way my desire to know every detail about a disease, because it is interesting to me, was often frustrated. I did not always get enough time to know the details, particularly in biochemistry and pharmacology. Time was always lacking. (2am26) Less valuable may be the fact that in these years I became more impatient with people who have little internal control and that I may be too easily irritated by that mentality now. (2af30) Least valuable was being in the first problem-based learning class and having to go through all that. (4am28)

New Mexico students, most in-state like Mercer's, and exhilarated by the curriculum like Hawaii's, also appreciate that faculty go out of their way to teach and that whole-person and preventive as well as standard medicine is taught. They prize their own camaraderie, diversity, and willingness to cooperate.

They speak with wonder about acquiring the knowledge and opportunity to practice medicine. New Mexico aims to humanize the specialist and generalist alike.

- There is a lot of enthusiasm at the school in each of the different phases of medical education. I take a good deal of satisfaction in seeing the growth in my own competence. I am now 29 weeks and 3 days away from gaining the MD degree. There is a great deal of camaraderie in my experience [here], a lot of support in studying. . . . On call some nights in the emergency room, it is very gratifying for me to communicate to other students about patients using the information and skills that I was taught. I like the commitment of faculty at the school of medicine. They are actually training students to be doctors. I look back and see the worth of what I have been taught. Faculty go out of their way to help students here. (4wm34)
- The pluses . . . include the diversity of the people [here] . . . the benefits from everyone's experiences and perspectives . . . the challenges for everyone in this. People also help each other learn, for example, in the gross anatomy cadaver lab. It seems each is able to teach the other. I like in general the give and take of each other's strength. This happens both among students and among faculty. I am also gratified with a certain dispelling of myths about Native Americans while I have been here. In general I think that many people are open-minded to the new perspective that Native Americans bring to the medical school. I am also satisfied with the structure of the traditional track. In the third year, there are opportunities to learn one-on-one from doctors in the wards. I have been learning to adapt and change in frequently changing situations in different rotations. I think this engenders self-confidence. Most of all, I appreciate how lucky I am to be who I am and where I am, the uniqueness of the role I am assuming, the deep satisfaction I have in being able to help others. (3nm28)
- I like best the nurturing environment for learning [here]. It reminds me a little of a child asking, "What is this? What is that?" And the parent answers! They do this for us here! I had never experienced education like this before. I

thought it was just the primary-care curriculum, but in the
third year I discovered that almost everyone here is excited
to teach if you are interested to learn. Compared to the
fourth-year students I have met from other schools, it is
like a family here. They give feedback not only on our
learning, whether is it adequate and so forth, but also on
our interpersonal skills, how we treat other people and are
treated by them. They emphasize learning and practicing
these skills over the years. This has helped me develop the
confidence to accept as normal skills that I have never been
taught before. It has redefined normal for me. We are also
taught here that it is okay to care about the whole person,
for example, whether they have the money to pay for their
care, wherever they live and so forth. I have learned that
traditionally trained fourth-year residents do not even
know how much drugs cost. They do not consider it their
business. There is also the fact that we get involved in the
community in a preventive and regular medicine way and
that this happens in the first year, in the first half of the
first year. They make learning fun here by taking away the
pressure of grades and by questioning how your whole
group does. You can pick up as many flowers as you want
here. (4wf35)

Several years into their practices, New Mexico students
imagine that they will have most benefited from having learned
how to learn.

- I will have become aware here of what I do not know and
  learned to feel comfortable with the fact that I do not have
  to know everything, because I can always learn. I will have
  learned here what is important. It will also be positive that
  I could continue my epidemiologic research interests.
  (4wm34) A positive will be just being out of school ...
  learning to do more, being able to apply facts to illness and
  people, having people appreciate what I can give, and all
  without being given a grade! I think it is a privilege to
  have medical skills. (3nm28) [It will be] knowing how to
  learn, not only recognizing what I do not know, but knowing where to go for what I need, not feeling fearful of what

I do not know. I will continue saying, "Okay, I do not know, will you show me how to do that?" . . . Another positive is knowing what you want to do. Because of the primary-care curriculum first-year clinical course, you discover whether or not you want family practice, primary care, rural community, or other specialties. [I: And you yourself?] I want to do dermatology (4wf35)

Yet complaints are registered by traditional and primary-care students alike, respectively, that the trees and that the forest are too much emphasized in the first two years. And a Native American and a female student each report incidents of discrimination.

- Improvements of problems around which the tutorials run and broader changes in curriculum at the school [are needed]. Mastery of the forest while learning the trees has been problematic for me. The trees have been easier than the forest. Yet the forest needs to be learned too and this does not always happen here. (4wm34) [For me it is] the obligation of having to learn certain materials within certain time constraints but not having the "big picture" or interconnections explained. I am also dissatisfied with having to learn details which do not seem tied to the reality of clinical practice. I [want] to learn what you really need to know to be a good doctor. Occasionally I have had to deal with subtle racist implications, for example, about affirmative action and how being a Native American I had presumably been accepted to the medical school on first application. It gets sort of tiring having to prove my worth. Some of this is due to an attitude among some faculty of, "Well, I went through it, so you have to go through it too." But it is a different medical landscape now than it was 40 years ago. AIDS, for example, and other such diseases. I worry about the chance that my career will be destroyed by my acquiring certain infectious diseases. (3nm28)
- I chose the primary-care curriculum because it offered the forest and the big picture that [some have] found wanting in the traditional curriculum. The primary-care curriculum is outstanding in terms of context, in terms of anat-

omy, physiology, disease process. But for us, the problem is
that we never get the trees! We must learn the trees on our
own, with little help. In my third year, I had to ask what a
split protein was! In the third year, you go back together
with the traditional-track students, then we help with the
big picture, and they help us with the details. Third- and
fourth-year students trained in the traditional track will
have difficulty in applying all the trees to clinical work, to
the point where it even costs them an extra year. This does
not happen if you see the big picture. Still, for the primary
care curriculum students, it is the trees that are the big minus. The general negative in the third year is how you are
treated by some people. It depends on the subspecialty, but
some people have very traditional attitudes and do not like
women or minorities in medicine and do not even like patients. I have not encountered much bias against women,
but in surgery there have been pointed sexual remarks
both about patients and about me from staff. But I loved
general surgery anyway. It was not very nurturing, it was
even really crass sometimes, but I found it tolerable and
even comical. (4wf35)

Several years into practice, primary-care curriculum students anticipate encountering problems with labeling and with
incongruency between their less-conventional medical education at New Mexico and more conventional residencies elsewhere.

* A negative could be the public's and my own colleagues'
  perception of me as a family-practice physician. But I think
  that training in family practice as a resident at New Mexico will be less of a problem than at other places, as far as
  image or labeling is concerned. (4wm34) The negative that
  I anticipate will have been my fear of the unknown ... of
  whether I will miss some important information. For mi-
  nuses, the big one for me will have been that because we do
  not have grades, and because of how residency programs
  are set up, trying to get into competitive residency programs is tough. You have very little on paper, no GPA, no
  class standings. I will have to learn to count on the derma-

tology people here for getting me my interviews. The primary-care curriculum program may be better, but it is not the way the whole system works yet. (4wf35)

Minnesota pours new wine from old wine skins—in novel clinical correlations to standard pathophysiology instruction—and the students like it very well. For this, one even reports appreciating his first-year drilling in biomedical science. Minneapolis and Duluth campus students both enjoy early exposure to patients, and third- and fourth-year students, in the clinical phase of a rather conventional curriculum, are relieved by long-anticipated opportunities for close-contact clinical instruction. Minnesota ages pretty well.

- The pathophysiology course in the second year was just superb. A clinician taught it and the lectures were excellent. If I could absorb everything said there, I could graduate the next day. I still go back to my notes. [I: Were there any tutorials in that course?] Yes, I loved them, especially when I prepared ahead of time. By the end of the year, I just quit going to lectures and just started preparing for these groups. There were so many hours of lectures. (4wf35) I agree that being taught pathophysiology by clinician practitioners who gave lectures was very good. There was real clarity of thought. Most of the physicians were excellent communicators. You do not find that as much among the basic scientists. (3wf34)
- At Duluth . . . there were so many things built into the program that integrated what we were learning. Only after a few months of classroom experience, in the first year here, there is a preceptorship in community family practice where you can relate to a practicing physician. That experience made me want to go back into the classroom to learn the basic science. It made the basic science a little more bearable. It boosted my motivation to learn. Then, here in Minneapolis in my clerkship rotations, whenever we have done patient bedside medicine with an attending physician, everything suddenly became so clear. It is so positive, so very positive—it is a gestalt-type thing. (3wm28) [In] the second-year preceptorship on the Duluth campus, three

times for 3 days each, I lived with a family-practice physician at the White Earth Indian Reservation. It was great to
see Native American people cared for as well as they were.
It reinforced what I wanted to do and what I intend to do
through the Indian Health Service. (3nm34)

- The pathophysiology course was strong, but it was also the
more effective for the basic-science courses that we took in
the first year. These were really drilled into us. There was a
lot of rote memorization out of textbooks in the first-year
basic-science courses. It hurt, it was painful, but I cannot
think of a better way to make pathology sink in than to
have this basic foundation. As for my clinical rotations in
the last few months, I think that we are lucky to have such
a strong network of affiliated hospitals. (3wf27) In Iran, I
had a rich sciences program at Alborz High School. Subsequently, I took many science courses and, by the time I entered medical school, I was very ready for doing medicine.
Here for me, the most important thing has been the integration of pathophysiology in the second year with clinical
medicine. Actually, that integration of science and clinical
medicine begins in the first year here. This is a high point
for me right now. (3wm25)

- Half of what I have most liked here is the chance to study
in small groups. That was the way it was for me in gymna-
sium as I prepared to study medicine in Poland. The other
half is the early clinical experience that you have here in
contrast to the European system where you can wait 6
years before you have exposure to clinical medicine.
(3wm29) I learn best in small groups with a mentor. For
this reason, I really enjoyed the third-year clinical rotations as well as my work so far in the fourth year. It has
been a really spectacular experience to work with staff.
They will give you a lot of time and they have taught me
very well. This is the kind of learning that I remember
best. It brings out the best in me. In cardiology, for example, one member of the department came in an hour early,
just to teach me and a resident to read EKGs [electrocardi-
ograms]. That was Doc McBride at Ramsey. The same thing
happens in other rotations too. (4wf38) I am in my second
year and the most positive thing for me to date has been

that clinical rotations for clinical medicine start at the end of the first year. I cannot believe I am here doing pediatrics at St. Paul's Hospital! We just saw a 9–year-old Turner syndrome! (2wm32)

What students anticipate appreciating most about Minnesota in retrospect is the mentoring and personal relations in clinics, the daily challenge of learning so much, acquiring knowledge for the long term, and the occasional instance in their conventional predoctoral education when self-directed learning was encouraged.

• The most helpful part will be to have gotten to know some clinicians on a personal basis and to have been working with them early on in the real world. (3nm34) [It will be] the mentor relationships that I had. (3wf27) [It] will have been . . . that medical school means an increasing amount of knowledge, the challenge of so much to learn. There are at least 20 or 30 things a day to learn! This has brought out the best in me. (3wm25) Most helpful will have been the fact that I found several physicians, for example, my advisor, who have been very helpful to me learning medicine through the back door, listening to their life stories, finding out about what is ahead. (3wm29) For me [it] will have been the whole opportunity to go to medical school in my 30s, just being able to do it, with the financial support system in place, not to mention the support of tutors, of a quarter off, of so much choice in the fourth-year system. There are problems, but in general there are very good support systems here. It is a very secure feeling once the horrible admissions process is over. (4wf38) Most helpful will have been learning how to study independently and to delineate what you need to know, which I learned especially in the pathophysiology courses. (2wm32) I will look back on one situation that summarizes it for me. I am very easily intimidated. Once an attending physician wanted me to grab a patient's thigh and do a knee-jerk reflex. The lesson was that I could touch his thigh. That attending really helped me to put down, or better, not to build barriers. (3wm28) Most valuable will have been the people I have

seen already who are continually learning, not stagnating,
searching for themselves. (3wf34) I already had a lot of experience and skills dealing with people. Therefore, the
most important will have been the content I learned. For
me, this mostly came in the second year, although some of
the principles from the first year were important too. What
I have gained is useful information for the long term.
(4wf35)

Complaints registered target Minnesota's standard educational matrix and include the reportedly liberal bias in the
teaching of ethics, a lack of legal and economic content in clinical courses, fragmentary basic science courses that employ too
many lecturers, sacrificing patient perspective to basic-science
content in instruction; spotty teaching by residents on wards,
and class bias in granting educational loans to enter primary-
care practice.

- The negative for me is in the teaching of ethics here. I am
  on the legal committee for the Minnesota Medical Association and I feel that there is a strong slant toward issues of
  the uninsured and advocacy from a socialist point of view. I
  think that more libertarian or utilitarian viewpoints tend
  to be omitted in the clinical-medicine course. I have been
  trained as a CPA and I do believe that an ethics content in
  courses is an obligation. My second complaint is that ethical discussion in the clinical-medicine course has occurred
  more on a philosophical plane. I think that it needs to be
  much more concrete. (2wm32) I think that more legal and
  economic issues should be taught in the clinical-medicine
  course. I think it is important to know how and what to
  document in daily notes in a medical practice. The subject
  of legal documentation, of libel, of issues of responsibilities
  and related issues have only come up so far in the psychiatry rotation! We need to know more about legal issues, cost
  control, and these practical subjects. (4wf38)
- About the basic sciences . . . I am used to being taught in
  small groups with passionate teachers who do not chase
  money. In the lecture format at Minnesota, for example, in
  biochemistry, there are too many professors. Each thinks

that his part is the most important, and there is no chance to interact. (3wm29)

- My complaint is that we were not taught patients' perspectives enough, so we wound up more with the scientific aspects of being a doctor. (3wm25) My only negative is the sporadic teaching I get from residents on the wards. I know that they are busy, and that is okay. They are hard-worked. But still, some are fantastic and some are not. Some are great at what they do and teach well, and some are just bitchy, overworked, and unavailable. (3nm34)

- They are trying very hard to get us to go into primary care here, but they are not offering incentives. I think that the federal government should support primary-care physicians. My debt now is $75,000, and I am in my third year. I cannot do primary care earning $50,000 or $60,000 a year and manage my debt. This encourages the upper-middle classes, which do not have access to the health professions loans at 5%, to go into subspecialty medicine. (3wf27)

- For me [it] was the admissions process. I found it degrading. Every school to which I applied told me that subjectively I was great but objectively I was a long shot. They told me this at Duluth too. I applied to 11 schools right out of college, and then to six the next year. I re-took the MCATs and then applied to three schools here in Minnesota. I improved my MCATs. They had me believing that I was not capable. (3wm28) My experience was similar. I applied to 45 schools the first year and to 36 the second year. Of these latter, 35 did not admit me because I was an exchange student with a student visa. (3wm29)

- Yes, it is hard to get in, and once you are here, you are a captive audience. You have to take it, even the lousy stuff, because there are so many who want into medical school. It relieves some faculty of the responsibility to be excellent. As a result, partly, the first 2 years are pretty poorly coordinated. Courses did not flow, for example, in coordinating the organ systems and the drugs courses. It is really just a bag of subjects here. Also, there are a lot who do not know how to teach here. Standing up in front of a class is only information dispensation. Thus there is a lot of notetaking from the oracle, of memorization. Even in the small groups,

I found that these, too, were into just dispensing, only in a smaller setting. Then too, there are examples where a lecture should begin at 8:00 a.m. and the lecturer shows up at 8:30 and just covers the 1 hour of material in 30 minutes. I remember that he was so excited that he had done it in 30 minutes, imparted all the information! And then the same thing happened at 9:00! (3wf34) I found that there were excellent teachers here along with the laundry-list makers. But there is an inconsistency in teaching across the 4 years. In the third and fourth years, I wanted teachers as good as the pathophysiology teachers, but I did not find them. I was ready to be interactive, but they did not have the time. They were just caught up in the mechanics of rotation. After second-year pathophysiology, I was not used to being taught like this. (4wf35)

In retrospect, Minnesota students imagine that they will least appreciate the honors (grading) system, subjectivity in grading, the way-too-many lectures, and the first 2 years' drudgery.

- The least helpful thing will have been the emphasis placed on striving for honors grades. The effect of the honors system is that you feel bad if you do not put a total effort into a rotation. There is always a twinge of guilt later on. (3wf27)
- Least helpful will have been the people who did not care or who stood in the way. For example, there was a person in the first day of my rotations who did not like my choice of neurosurgery. He was a psychiatrist. He always left me out of all the question-and-answer discussions. (3wm25) Least helpful will have been the whole idea of struggling to achieve grades when in fact these were not determined by objective measurement but by someone's judging you on the basis of specialties. It happens all the time, the subjective part of evaluation, measuring performance very imperfectly. There should be more specific criteria. (3wm29) Least helpful will have been ... an enormous loan debt, about $100,000. The average here is $60,000. We need different funding people to talk about alternative sources that do not take 3 weeks to write the applications for. (4wf38)

Least helpful will have been the lectures. I do not go to lectures. I do not find them helpful. (2wm32) Least helpful will have been the experience of going through the board exams. Why on earth should we do these? I was palpitating! (3wm28) Least helpful will have been a lot of drudgery in the first 2 years. I worked very hard for good grades and most of it evaporated out of my head after the exams. Most of what was taught in this context was irrelevant. (3wf34) Least helpful will have been a lot of the first-year stuff. (4wf35)

Above all, Case Western Reserve's students appreciate the company that the school's distinct admissions policy allows them to keep. They enjoy their own diversity and willingness to help one another, the tradition of independent learning, curricular flexibility, early exposure to patients, and faculty dedication to teaching. Case Western Reserve maintains its students' confidence because it maintains confidence in its students.

- Most positive for me has been the process of learning, learning from, learning with, and learning through my peers, my classmates, and the house staff. This has been the most consistently sustaining and rewarding part for me. You are exposed to a wide range of people here and inescapably you are obligated to work with many different types. This has been a very challenging experience for me. [And] I have enjoyed the patient exposure from the first year following in this curriculum. My exposure in the first year prepared me well for the wards. I felt comfortable with establishing rapport and establishing boundaries. If you hit the third year and you are unable to work with people, it shows and it makes the experience unpleasant. It is not written anywhere that the hospital has to be an alienating place. You cannot teach this, but you can expose people to it and provide an atmosphere. I had great role models. (4wm27)
- For me [it] was the early exposure to patients, for example, through the baby program under the medical apprenticeship program. I also enjoyed all the electives. Both of these helped me keep my learning tangible. There are a thou-

sand ways to gain exposure to patients at Case Western Reserve. I am not here to pass the national boards at the highest level. I like people. This is the reason that I came to Case Western Reserve. My stepmother graduated from the medical school here. She was 32 when she applied and she applied from Africa when she was in the Peace Corps. These are the kinds of people that the medical school attracts. (2wf24)

- I have most liked the patient contact [and] would have liked even more contact in the first 2 years. I would have also liked more time in the second 2 years to study for integration. This could be taken much further here, even considering as much as I got. I have treasured it. I also [like] the flexible schedule but wonder if that too could not be expanded. During my second year, I stopped going to a lot of classes and started learning on my own. I do better with choices. I found that 5 hours of class is too much. On-the-job learning really works for me. I have also liked the way we teach each other here. We taught each other basic science. There is a real camaraderie. I have liked working in teams, for example, with the nurses on the wards. (4wf44) The atmosphere is less competitive at Case Western Reserve. People are freer to work with other people. (4wf36) We do not get ranked and there is a scheduling of classes that helps for getting together. (4wf44) In my entire 4 years here, I have heard a test score mentioned from a student only once. (4wm27) I would add that I was not as lucky as some, but I did get one clinical teacher who liked to teach, and my learning curve went way up then. When you get the one that works, it is really amazing. (4wf44)

- For me [it] has been my relationship with faculty. Anytime I had trouble in a subject, faculty were willing to help. For example, in histology, they would tutor you. The same was true in neurology and in the neuroanatomy course. There was a review session every week. "I will stay up all night," my instructor would say, "if it helps you get the material." I have also liked the flexibility of the curriculum, that classes are from 8:00 until 12:00 noon. This is important because I had the rest of my time free. (2bm23) Of course, the drawback to this is Saturday classes! (2wf24) I had been working as a nurse for over 10 years. I chose Case Western Reserve. It was the only application that I made for early decision. I knew the flexibility of the schedule, the morning classes 6 days a week. The other thing I knew was the elective part of the curriculum and the early exposure to patients. Having been a nurse, it would have made me nuts just to be in class. I knew that at any medical school I could get the basic information, but here I could work part-time during the first 2 years and could find time to work with my son. (4wf36)

Several years into practice, Case Western Reserve students imagine that they will have most benefited from the school's trademark encouragement of the individual.

• I have not had a traditional focus in healing, yet I feel that I am accepted here because of my beliefs, or possibly despite them. I am very grateful for the accepting atmosphere at Case Western Reserve. I was a potter before I came and I have studied holistic and alternative therapies. I view myself as a bridge between these ideas and Western medicine. (4wf44) The legacy for me of Case Western Reserve . . . will be that I was allowed to be myself . . . have a life . . . pursue what I was interested in . . . fly where I wanted to fly. The experience of being allowed to grow now will allow me to do so in the future. I can be the kind of physician I want to be. I am accepted for who I am. This gives me the confidence to practice the art of medicine, the confidence to be creative. (4wf36) I am interested in teaching and, because of my experience here, I will have a real understanding of students' needs. I will know that you do not have to bash students to get them to learn. I will be a more empathetic teacher. (2bm23) For me [it] will be in my perspective, in an appreciation of the strains and limitations of medical science, and in how I will take care of my patients. I will categorically refuse to somaticize everything or chase lab tests. (4wm27) Case Western Reserve will have enhanced my empathy for the patient and the student. The people process has been emphasized here, the dealing with the entire patient and the family, not just the acute care of an illness. (2wf24)

Honoring their school in the breach, Case Western Reserve students challenge the sequencing of courses, organ-based teaching approach, and learning geared to independent, not external, standards. They want better preparation in pharmacology and anatomy for national boards, on which a particularly poor performance was recently turned in. They object, as at Mercer, to the second-class treatment of clinic patients, and they chafe at curricular rigidity.

- I think that there should be a major re-haul of the first 2 years. These are too intellectually exclusive of the real-life experience. There is so much brain work and sitting alone. You are thrown into the second 2 years without knowing very much what is expected. All 4 years should be more the same, should be more integrated. (4wf44) In the Case Western Reserve organ-system method of teaching, they divide cardiovascular into a first-year and a second-year course. I had trouble waiting for the pathology part in the second year. My boyfriend got both the first year. He is in a discipline-based program. I am impatient to learn. I would like all the cardiology during the first year, the normal and the pathological all at once to complete the cycle. (2wf24) I have not liked the way patients are divided into staff patients and private patients. [I: Do you mean the social class aspect?] Yes, and the way procedures are done, allowed to be done, on the staff patients by the less-experienced people. The private patients do not get this "doctor versus patient" syndrome. (4wm27)
- In pharmacology, they should emphasize more teaching about drugs. They are not doing as good a job teaching us about drugs. (2bm23) We get drug dynamics and theory, but we do not know any drugs in particular, and for the national boards we are getting scared about this. (2wf24) We have a reputation for this, and the same is true in anatomy. (4wf44) [I: What do you think the effect will be on the curriculum in coming years of about a quarter of second-year students having failed the boards last year?] They will not

change the organ-based approach, but they will enhance pharmacology. They will have students remember 200 to 300 drugs for the boards and there will be more board-type questions throughout the first 2 years. (2bm23) In general, there is already now an environment in which students want to be taught toward an external measure. The recent national boards experience may dilute and destroy the curriculum here. It could be gutted. Students will just realize that you can take a Kaplan course, just as you can do at any of the 125 medical schools in the country. If this happens, the marginal value of Case Western Reserve will disappear. (4wm27) I disagree. I think that Case Western Reserve will hold the line. (4wf44) But people want their tickets punched. There is a market out there and they will change Case Western Reserve or go elsewhere. There is a big debate in the student community whether Case Western Reserve should embrace the boards as a mandatory exercise or not. (4wm27) I agree with the point about pharmacology and about anatomy. Case Western Reserve students are well-known for lacking in these subjects. I personally have not had much trouble with pharmacology because when I came I had used medicines for years. I am an RN in critical care and emergency nursing. The other thing is that I am not probably a typical student and I would like more flexibility in the electives program to orient people to patient care. Case Western Reserve recruits for prior life experience. If some of this experience has been clinical, then the elective system should be more flexible. (4wf36)

But at Case Western Reserve, as at Mercer, the positive prevails even in what students imagine will appear to have least benefited them.

- It may be that a couple of years out of Case Western Reserve I will have less of a knowledge base compared to my peers, but, 4 or 5 years out of the program, it will not be an issue. (2wf24) I think that I will have missed some aspects of the basic sciences from the point of view of my first years out of medical school. (2bm23) I do not think that I will be lacking anything. I think that many with whom I will come in contact will wish that they had come here to medical school. I also want to say ... that doctors should go to nursing school first, before medical school. Nursing is a totally different methodology. Doctors and nurses should know how the other is educated. (4wf36) I do not think that there is anything that I will regret in 7 or 8 years. (4wm27) I do not think that I will regret anything, either. I am getting what is best for me here. (4wf44)

Dartmouth's tough curriculum plainly puts students through extreme stress, even as they acknowledge hard-won competence. The school is rugged enough, apparently, that positive recollections are limited—left to having to run an emergency room in West Africa, having refused to adopt a victim mentality in the early going, and having taken an exceptional course late in the program.

- It is difficult to find a primary positive. I do recognize that I am slowly accumulating knowledge and competence in areas that I want desperately to be competent in and to offer to people. This is apparent to me in fits and starts and at odd moments. In tutoring for example, when I am able to help fellow medical students understand a concept, and when I can understand a disease process, when I can think it through. Thus the big black hole is beginning to fill a little bit. I did not prepare for medical school as an undergraduate. I have done well, but it was a tough switch. (2wf28)
- I had a positive experience in the fourth year when I received a fellowship through Beth Israel Hospital to go to Gabon, West Africa, for 3 months, in charge of a 30–bed ward of children. It was so good to get away. I ran the emergency room. The fourth year here is a tremendous break from the torture of medical education. Very positive things happen. Brains turn on again. For example, there were six of us in Jonathan Ross's course in advanced internal medicine. It is the best course here, maybe ever! He teaches effectively. We teach second-year medical students physical diagnosis. It is an opportunity to review and to share mate-

rial. There are 4 days of decision analysis and 1 day of teaching second-year students each week. It is the only course here that teaches you how to think. It completely changes the way you think about medical care. You apply statistical techniques to case studies and you learn where decision ends and value judgment begins. The course convinced me that medical education is not a fantasy. So, yes, the first year is tremendously challenging. It is a very destructive year. In some ways it was so bad that a very important thing happened for me. I soon figured out that if I wanted to survive as a person, I had to make a break from feeling like a victim to defining a clear sense of myself. I went through a long period of solitude and struggle. I grew a great deal in the process, but I have seen it work out badly for others. (4wm26)

- My best course was . . . an elective, medicine for the underserved. It is 80% student-driven, for no credit, and speakers are student sponsored. I have also had opportunities to do electives elsewhere, for example, in Rhode Island and in Cooperstown, New York. (4wm31)

Only one Dartmouth student interviewed finds even faint praise, looking back from her imagined future practice.

- If I can get through this [medical education] experience, one thing that I will enjoy in retrospect is that I am now being presented with a tremendous amount of material. There is something positive in looking at some of this excess. A lot should be taken out. The positive thing is that there is a hell of a lot of useful material that we are learning. (2wf28)

Grievances cascade at Dartmouth, all connected by how little student-centered the curriculum comes across. Medical educators of every persuasion should listen closely to these strikingly clear calls.

- The most difficult thing for me has been going from the position of competent professional before medical school into the role of student again, medical student. Before, I worked

in pediatric medicine as a research associate on the psychosocial part. I had a patient population, peers, and so forth
. . . at Children's Hospital in Washington, D.C. It was amazing . . . the discrepancy between what I had been and what
I am now. My problem in switching roles is really given in
the nature of the beast, [but] I did not anticipate it. I cannot pinpoint why I was so thrown by the curriculum. So it
is hard to know how to change it. But one thing that I do
feel strongly about is that, while I came with a lot of enthusiasm to learn this material, after less than a month it was
gone! There must be a better way to capitalize on this kind
of enthusiasm. I moved mountains to get here, to get into
medical school. I tried and I did it. I do not understand why
my energy could not have been capitalized on, even engendered. I was dreaming of something more like an apprenticeship that I would learn from a mentor in relationships
of shared enthusiasm. [I: Any of these to date?] Yes, but not
in the classroom. Class roles threaten the mentor relationship. There is a study in the psychological literature, I remember it, that if you take children who are spontaneously
artistic and you reward them for it and then you remove
that reward, then they will stop drawing. In a way that is
what has happened to me despite myself here. There is
something extremely impersonal about this whole medical
education. Oddly, wanting to do it is very personal in contrast. But that personal is externalized in an instant, the
moment you start the process here. Ideally, what I would
do, my remedy, would be to go back to the old system of four
to six people in a room with an anatomist. In the old system there was teamwork and cooperation. There was little
objective evaluation. When I came, I knew that I was coming to an auditorium and a lecture hall, but I did not anticipate the personal ramifications of that. In fact the well-
roundedness of many of the students here may contribute
to some of the difficulties that we experience. Dartmouth
sets this up by its admissions policy. The sad thing is that
it is not facilitated by the curriculum, which is impersonal,
deadening, hard to understand. Let me give one example,
the clinical symposia course. It is supposed to touch psychosocial issues in medicine, but we were actually given a set

of rules of how to behave in telling patients that they were dying. We were taught that it would be better to be impersonal and that people should avoid talking about their own experience with pain, that this would break the necessary barrier between sickness and the doctor role. I could not disagree more. I just know that it is better that I admit when I do not really know what to do or fully understand something. I know that a growing knowledge of myself will better guide me than any rules on how to tell a person that they are dying. (2wf28)

- I too came with a lot of prior life experience [and] found the first year extremely dramatic. The course load was 8 hours of lectures a day, with only Tuesday and Thursday afternoons off. Anatomy was devastating, just sitting in that classroom. I was a firefighter. I used to jump from helicopters and that sort of thing. I had been out there, really. I have been through a lot. But I can tell you that the first year here was pure hell. I kept hearing about the rationale, that it was to bronze us, that it was a kind of hazing. But whatever they want to call it, it was awful. The positive for me was a couple of classmates, one in particular. If she had quit then I would have quit. Then later, you look forward to a course, for example, community medicine or epidemiology, but the faculty does very little with it and you get very little positive feedback. For the most part, at Dartmouth, you learn for test-taking only, not because it is an interesting subject. (4wm31) It is a sad day when you have to stop trying to relate what you are learning in class to what you want to do with your life. And I think that there are more people at risk than [it appears]. For example, I would be willing to bet that people would identify me as sailing through at the very times when I was struggling the most, at the lowest point in my life, which was until Christmas of the first year. (2wf28) Last year, in my third year, working through the clerkships I recall that the grade was always present as well. I was always there until 4:00 a.m. and received little positive feedback. The only positive was the people and the patients. (4wm31) [I: It seems that Dartmouth has miles to go in terms of student-centered learning?] Yes. (All.) [I: How would you remedy it?] The remedy that one of us adopted was just not to come to class for 18 months. (4wm31) Instead, I learned everything in my room.

I never really went through the second year. (4wm26) I went to class out of fear of what I was missing. (4wm31) If I had gone to class, I would have failed because in class I could not follow the lecture and it was a waste of time. I followed the maxim, Why learn by day what you can learn by night? (4wm26) But your class's experience, the class of 1993, was infamous. (2wf28) Yes, they butchered the class of 1993. We started on the first day with seven courses, including biochemistry, histology, anatomy, embryology, neuroanatomy, community medicine, genetics. Seven different exams! (4wm26) We started with three. Gross anatomy, microanatomy, and clinical symposium. (2wf28) But we went through it without deriving any pride at all, so the hazing failed. (4wm31) [I: Why did they change the curriculum between your 2 years?] Because everyone was so shaken by what happened. So many did not make it. One of the women who had to repeat the first year had actually climbed Mount Everest! [I: How does the new dean figure into this?] (4wm26) He came in between our first and second years. We told him point blank. We called a meeting with him and told the truth. We met to welcome him and told him straight. The next week he cut down classes by 20%. This was July 1990. He became our hero in a sense. And he said, "Cut 10% more for the next year or two." (4wm31) Our syllabus was a little choppy because of the change. (2wf28) It was the old guard faculty who pushed for so much content in the curriculum. The curriculum committee was always the arena in which to fight for your turf. (4wm26) [I: How could there be more role modeling, mentoring at Dartmouth? Should it be more formalized?] Not necessarily formalized, but better publicized as a goal, agreed upon by people acting as mentors. (2wf28)

- Medical school was brutal for me, especially the first 2 years. I had to work extremely hard to pass all the time. There was just a huge amount of material. I had 8 hours of lecture every day and the test-taking pressure pushed me to my complete limits. Yet at the same time, my brain was shut off in order to get through it. My second week here, doing immunology—I had done a lot before coming to Dartmouth—a professor said something in class that was very dated. I told him so, but he was not interested at all. I decided then to keep my mouth shut. There are a number of people who I know who have suffered a great

deal here. In my class, 8 to 12 people out of 80 were not promoted into the second year, about 15%. In one course, the clinical symposium, which is designed to teach a variety of psychosocial issues in medicine, including the doctor–patient
relationship, although I had looked forward to it incredibly, I
found it infuriating that the faculty did nothing with this incredibly important subject. Personal friends, not at Dartmouth, were very supportive and important to me, also my god-
father, who is a physician. (4wm26)

Images of how future medical practice will benefit from
past medical education are no less gripping at Dartmouth.

• I will recall how we have been tested in the minutia and
the trivia. I will recall how I had to choose between learning material and passing tests, how I passed the tests and
[some] did not, how [some] read the books and I did not. I
remain very skeptical about curriculum change at Dartmouth. There may be some change, but what, I feel, needs
to change are attitudes as much as class hours. These do
not change quickly and I doubt that it will be a very different educational experience 5 years from now. I think that
many medical students who have not had any independent
experience before coming to medical school are not aware
that they are being abused. They study all week and Saturday they party and Sunday they wake up and go back to
work and perform well and so forth. (4wm26) I will recall
how board-driven all of us were. It is an incredible alba-
tross. In the new-directions committee, we talk about core
material and skills and very exciting things, and then, I
just remember the coming board exam. Medical school here
is really a college experience in a sense. For me, a mentor
sharing his experiences would change everything. It would
be very important to put students in positions where they
have some control, even if they do not always understand
what they are doing. (2wf28)

Harvard's New Pathway is appreciated by students for the
independence, personal and intellectual, that it affords them, its
orientation to patients, method training in how to reason medi-

cally, the first 2 years' learning how to learn, mutual support and sharing among students, and the ambience in tutorials.

- I came to Harvard because of the curriculum, the New Pathway. For me, the positive has been being able to focus on what I am interested in academically. If you are not interested in something, then you learn the basics but do not have to spend a lot more time on it. I also like being taught how to think about patients as well as science. And I appreciate the flexibility that you have to be as diligent or nondiligent a student as you want. Thus I have also enjoyed having time with my husband too. I have made the choice not to be a top student, to have a life in medical school as well. Had I been at a more traditional school, I'd have suffocated. I have also appreciated the patient–doctor course on the whole. It helped me feel comfortable by the end of the first year to walk into a room and interact with a patient, even though we don't learn physical examination until the second year. Four to 5 years out of training I imagine that I will be working full-time, but less than a ridiculous schedule, in child psychiatry, preferably in private practice, but probably for an HMO. (2wf25)
- I chose HMS also because of the New Pathway. I wanted the flexibility [and] liked having the School of Public Health nearby. I am just coming off taking the boards the last 2 days. The last section was especially brutal for me. I felt incompetent. I never studied so hard for feeling so unprepared. There were so many facts and details that I hadn't learned. I have a friend at Tufts who, before the boards, worried that, in lectures on histamine regulators, second-messenger systems had only been mentioned a few times. Not one of my lectures mentioned them!, I thought. Yesterday, that was the negative of the school for me, that it had not prepared me for the boards. Today, it's the flipside. I am through and they are finished. Now, I ask, would I have wanted the first 2 years designed around these exams? Last week I would have said, yes. Now, no. The boards are unpleasant, but talking with friends at other medical schools, I know that here I have been taught how to think about questions. I feel very comfortable about this, about

how the curriculum is designed around this. In these 2
years I have always felt that I was in the ball park. At
some point I know that it will not be sufficient. But for the
first and second years it is what I wanted, and this place
has done that. Four years out of training, I will be in internal medicine with training in clinical epidemiology. I may
be doing clinical research but I will be active seeing patients too. (2am23)

- I am from Montreal . . . I am almost 29 . . . I chose Harvard
for the same reasons others have expressed, the same reasons for which I applied to McMaster and Case Western Reserve. For me, it is the lack of competitiveness among peers
here. For every exam I have taken, I have had some kind of
study group, friends helping friends, sharing. There has
been no possessiveness of knowledge at all. [All: Yes.] It
cannot be overstated how great that is. It feels like we are
colleagues already helping each other, consulting. (1wf28)
But this changes in the third year when the honors program comes in and people start competing for specialties,
knowing that only about 10% will get high honors. Then it
is not as cozy as the first 2 years. (3wm30) Just discovering
Medline was also very positive for me. I love the time allowed in this program for students to pursue their own interests. I have done a literature search, for example, on cer-
vical cancer, scanning for how viral proteins interact with
P53 tumor suppressor genes. I imagine having a joint residency in psychiatry and internal medicine someday and
work of some sort with psychosomatic illnesses. (1wf28)

- I am a third-year student, 30 years old, from Iowa. I have a
BA from Harvard in general biology. It was my fourth major, which I just managed to complete before graduation. I
worked for the Boston Consulting Group after graduating,
then went into the Peace Corps for 3 years, in Swaziland. I
had had such good experiences here in college [that] I
would have come even if there had been no New Pathway.
In the first 2 years, I liked the freedom to choose how I was
going to learn a given subject, and I was relieved to find
that I was well enough prepared for the third year, that I
did not have to relearn everything, that I knew how to
learn. The important thing about the first and second years

here was exposure to the mechanism of basic sciences, the hooks on which to remember things for the clinical years. We learned in broad strokes in the first 2 years, and that made some of us wary. But you then learn that you are expected to keep learning on the wards, to keep returning to your books, and this is what the first 2 years teach, persistence, creativity, literature searching. The second 2 years are difficult enough. You are shaped up by them. You have to keep learning, even if there is something that you did not exactly get the year before. When you don't know something in the third year, you look like a fool and you go home at night and relearn it. You go back to it. Here, you are definitely primed to a life-long cycle of learning. I will be an orthopedic surgeon, back in the Midwest or West, though not the coast. I like New Mexico very much. I will be in a private group practice. And I want to work from time to time overseas in clinics. Within orthopedics, I am interested in sports medicine. (3wm30)

- I had had some experience with [tutorials] before at Northwestern. I enjoyed the freedom there and here. I don't believe in forcing a body of knowledge. I fall asleep in lectures, really. I cannot get motivated to study for exams. I need academic and intellectual freedom. The only thing that gets me going is taking risks in learning, following leads. This is what I have appreciated here so far. I am 21, and a first-year student. I knew I wanted medicine for a long time and I knew I wanted Harvard because of the medicine, science, and technology program, though I am not in it now. I have no idea what I'll be doing 4 or 5 years after training. I'll see about biotechnology, public health, using my engineering background. Academic medicine is a possibility. I want to travel a lot. (1am21)

- I am first-year, 23, from Charlotte, North Carolina. Looking at Harvard, Yale, North Carolina, and New York schools, I thought Boston would be friendlier and I liked Harvard's name. I would have come just for that. But I also liked the time that classes ended each day under the New Pathway! Four years out of training, I imagine I will be in charge of a community health center in a rural part of the South, though that may change. I could work for the National Health Service Corps. The best part of my medical education to date has been the tutorial groups, how they work. There is conflict yes, but they usually work. I like the questions asked, thinking through ideas. People are receptive to my questions for the most part. I had a few courses set up like this before Harvard, but definitely not to this extent. (1bf23)

Harvard students imagine that, several years into practice, they will most appreciate having learned to balance the personal and professional, the chance to explore their medical interests, to actively question their instructors, and to be life-long learners prepared to interact with experts without fear.

- I imagine that I will most appreciate the ability to prioritize what I will have learned in these years between my professional and personal lives. You can learn to balance these in this program. (2wf25) I will appreciate the opportunities I had to discover how medicine works, to do a variety of things in my medical education, to discover that I am really interested in research and clinical research, for example. I will also like having taken three School of Public Health courses, society and health, human rights, and the pharmaceutical industry. I have been like a kid in a candy store here. (2am23) This is a school that welcomes questioning, likes people to rock the boat. You are received well when you go to people with questions. They let you run without interference. The approach is, "Good, question me." It is very alive. (1wf28) I imagine that I will most appreciate how I was taught the basic sciences. I really believe that we will have to go on learning, constant learning no matter what. In orthopedic surgery there are changes all the time. Laparoscopic, video surgery was not around 10 years ago. Who knows what it will be in 10 more years? I will appreciate the culture of creativity and change in learning that I learned. (3wm30) I will appreciate what will have been a liberal medical education. As a doctor trained this way, I can walk into any conference room—in public health, hospital, business settings—and be comfortable, talk, interact, because here you meet people, people

who are exciting and dynamic, and you learn how to interact. You lose the fear. (1am21)

But they also wonder whether tutorial instruction will
equip them with sufficient medical knowledge, and they object
to the pace and antiseptic, nonmedical tenor of basic-science lectures, the pedagogical noncorrespondence between New Pathway and later clinical instruction, and the uneven quality and
commitment of tutors. As at problem-based Mercer, however,
where students harbor similar uncertainties, Harvard students
find much to appreciate even in detailing program shortcom-
ings.

- I am always wondering whether it is working, whether I
  am getting it in tutorial. Everyone thinks about this. Also,
  the structure of some of the blocks, pharmacology, for
  example, in 3½ weeks, is frustrating in allowing so little
  time. The lectures are good, organized, competent, but it is
  all taught so fast with no time to come back to anything.
  (1bf23)
- What hasn't worked for me is that they are not motivating
  us, pointing us well enough in the direction of what medicine is all about. Most lectures in 2 hours do not get across
  a sense of what medicine is. They are trying to teach us too
  much. They fail to include the proper material in a fore-
  shortened period of time. I want a bit of motivation from
  lectures. I want a lecturer to say, "This is how you approach the topic, now go out and get the books and see
  whether you can do it." I want frame-of-mind stuff. Most
  lectures don't do this. Therefore I have to find it in tutorial.
  I have had great tutorial leaders. I have been lucky.
  (1am21)
- The downside in the second 2 years is that you are learning
  mostly from residents and attendings who have not gone
  through the learning process that you have. So you ask a
  resident a question and you want them to make it a task
  for the next day, a learning exercise, the way you were
  taught the first 2 years, but instead you get either no feedback at all or ridicule. Still, with our kind of learning becoming more widespread, the situation is likely to improve

gradually on the wards. I had one chief resident recently who stopped everything and taught us. She made a beautiful clay reconstruction of the internal structure of the entire female pelvis! It was really impressive, and I learned a great deal from her. I would want more of this sort of learning in the clinical years, and more applied instruments of assessment, problem sets. Traditional methods are fine, only I would like less of it. (3wm30)

- For me the negative is in the culture of teaching at Harvard, the emphasis on research as opposed to clinical medicine and on patients. For example, one lecturer was talking about the different drugs for treating Parkinson's disease and for treating depression. "We have rationally designed drugs for treating Parkinson's," he said, plainly satisfied. Yet people still die! I thought. When it came to depression, however, he was clearly frustrated by the fact that we have drugs for it that work but that we don't precisely understand! The point is that we are being taught for the most part by people with this perspective. We are not being trained to be doctors from the start here. Someone else said that they wanted motivation, not just information, from lectures, and I agree. I want to learn from people who understand suffering and how to treat it. For another example, 3 days ago, describing a study of diphtheria, the lecturer said offhand, "Now, for those of you actually interested in patients . . ." (1wf28)

- I agree that lectures are too research- and not enough patient-oriented. We are taught no compassion, too little sense of who we are, where we are, what we need to get out of the lectures. I need more context in order to understand. The lectures in pharmacology, for example, were wonderful, but much of it went right over our heads. Still, I will say that lecturers and course directors here are also open to criticism and to improving. Clearly, the strength of this curriculum is that it is willing to change constantly. (2am23) The course evaluations are very thick. (1wf28) And they give them to you to fill out the day of the final! (1bf21) But there is also a feedback lunch halfway through every block that all faculty come to. (1wf28) As a matter of fact, in the gastrointestinal and renal block, faculty sat there as

we ripped them apart. I was amazed at the level of respon-
siveness. We were very harsh. They listened, and it
changed in the next block and was done better. We actually
got respect. (2am23)

- There are obviously some professors who do and do not buy
into the New Pathway, and their in-fighting is very unpleasant. At the end of the physiology course, for example,
one lecturer said, "If you do not learn it now, you will get it
later." Another objected, "No, that's not true." This was in
the same room, just before the final! Also, in the course of
tutorials, they want us to focus on the psychosocial issues,
so much so that it almost becomes a joke, which creates a
backlash, considering that you may not have learned the
science yet. (2wf25) Some tutors support thinking through
the psychosocial stuff as long as it does not get in the way,
but you usually do not have to prepare, and there are no
readings. (1bf23) It is very tutor-driven. It is amazing how
much one tutor can shape things. (1wf28) Yes, there is wide
variability in tutors. (2wf25) In general there is a failure to
emphasize that the psychosocial makes a better, not just
nicer, doctor, a more efficient clinician. This is a failure
here of leadership, not just of individual tutors. It starts
with the course directors, and because of this there is variability at the tutorial level. (2am23) This applies to the patient–doctor course too. (2wf25)

Several years into practice, Harvard students imagine that
they will least appreciate the basic-science content that they
had to learn; the limited student-body diversity in terms of age,
race, and medical vocation; the narrowing of perspective due to
an ambience of ambition, academic research, and medical technique; their financial indebtedness at graduation and the restrictions it will have subsequently imposed; and a sense of having wasted time shooting in the dark.

- I will least appreciate the content of the basic sciences that
I learned. It will have been less important than the process.
(2wf25) I can't think of anything I will not appreciate.
(2am23) What I will regret is probably the lack of other
older students. It has been quite an isolating experience for

me. It would be a problem anywhere, I imagine, except Case Western Reserve. Here there are only five women in my class who are older than me. (1wf28) The downside is the cost, the debt I am coming out with. It definitely worries me, at about $100,000, and it will affect how I play out my career. I would like to be freer later on, say, to go do orthopedic surgery in Tanzania. As it is there will be something hanging over my head. (3wm30) I will regret having wasted a lot of time in the process, the feeling that I am not getting the most out of my time, that I am only shooting in the dark, not learning immense amounts of material. (1am21) My biggest regret will be wondering whether my medical education was worth it in terms of the debt. (1bf23)

• I will also regret that the diversity of people was not what I wanted in terms of what I am interested in, like community clinics, working with people. Here it is mostly high-tech clinical medicine and research. I worry that I will be out in a community with very different needs. Being a woman of color has not been an issue for me at Harvard any more or less than it would have been elsewhere. There has been nothing tangible, no one saying anything specifically. But some of my girl friends have been questioned in tutorial, questioned about their knowledge base, whether they really know their basic sciences. Then there is the idea of affirmative action. But it is not generally discussed. (1bf23) Is it color or gender? (2wf25) Some of both, I'm sure. But the subtle things are pertinent, and you are bound to be a little paranoid in this culture anyway. (1bf23) It also sounds like a lack of shared interests. (1wf28) It is both. The more black students, the more interest there would be in community medicine. (1bf23) It is similar to my own lack of peers. The more older students, the more interest there would be in psychosocial issues. (1wf28) Yes, there are a lot of pressures here that send people in a traditional direction, a lot of ambitious people, a lot of debt, and the Harvard name. (1bf23) At Harvard, you can never know when you have done your best, when you have done enough. You can never be or do enough. If you are clinically oriented, then always there is all the academic research, the new drugs, techniques, and so forth. (1wf28)

Despite space constraints University of California, San Francisco (UCSF), offers a spacious kind of instruction that, by most accounts, students like very much, also because it is first-rate and, compared to the best private schools, cut-rate. Teachers teach well, reportedly, and students learn as well. Curricular flexibility is offered and widely accepted. Joint degrees and fifth years dot the landscape and the first-year pass–fail option reduces stress. UCSF gives public medical education a very good name.

- For me it is that I will graduate from a prestigious medical school which gives me leverage for future plans. This was my number one reason for coming here. My choices were Stanford and the University of California, Los Angeles, Irvine, or San Francisco. I chose UCSF because it is a public institution. I believe in public institutions, and UCSF was a cut above UCLA and Stanford. (4hf30) For me the primary positive has been the learning environment. Here you are safe to express your opinions. I had no prior medical background and therefore I have felt slower than most. Here it is okay to ask questions, to be wrong, and I am hypersensitive about being wrong. I am the type to not raise my hand for fear of being wrong. I had a choice between Harvard and UCSF. I chose UCSF because of the lesser expense and because I did not want to have a residency based on incurred debt. I have had no financial help from my family or my husband. (2wf23)
- The primary positive for me has been the faculty and the excellent teaching that I have had. It is the approach to teaching here. In the first 2 years I had some amazing teachers. Some of them have been hired specifically to teach ... and do not have to do research. I took my first year off too. It was important personal time. It was time to reflect about what I wanted to do. In that year I took an MPH [Master of Public Health] at UC Berkeley in maternal and child health. I also learned kayaking and hiked a 14,000–foot peak near Bishop, California. I like the fact that evaluations are taken very seriously here and often solicited. This is a place where strong praise is given ... particularly in the first 2 years, more sporadically in the third

and fourth years. (4wf31) I have liked the flexibility in terms of extending the curriculum. You can take an extra year. I went to Taiwan for 2 months and Beijing for 2 months and traveled for 5 months. Thirty to 40% of us take an extra year. That is why in my year there would be 180 instead of 140 graduating. It is not hard to get the administration to agree. It is easy to arrange. (4am27)

- The number one positive for me is the pass–fail system. I found it helpful once I started the program. It makes initially competitive people able to mix and interact better. Pass–fail helps to produce an environment of cooperation. It means that you choose how much you will push yourself, measuring yourself against yourself. (3wm24)

UCSF students, like Case Western Reserve's, imagine that several years into practice, they will most appreciate the school's having prompted them to pursue their own goals and to serve their own purposes, exposed them to a wide variety of fellow students and patients, and given them role models suited to their own individuality.

- Ten years hence, the primary positive of my medical education will be that it gave me the credential to do things that I believe in, like fighting for access to health care and being a role model for people in the community. (4hf30) To me [it] will be that it gave me an experience of a great diversity of students for those years. In this way I will understand culture better and better serve patients with different backgrounds. It will have been especially in small groups, where someone was interested in Chinese herbal medicine, or something, that I most experienced this diversity. (2wf23) My main positive 10 years hence will be that, because of its reputation, UCSF will have given me a ticket to do what I wanted to do. I do not like labels like Yale, UCSF, Peace Corps, but it will matter. It will be something of an achievement to have gone to UCSF. (4wf31) [Mine] will be that I was exposed to a tremendous amount of things, that I feel privileged and honored to be taking care of people, that I could not be doing it without having gone to medical school. About UCSF specifically, it will be that I learned medicine in conjunction with a wide variety of different patients, a very diverse patient population. I will also say that I was able to find role models, including a Chinese psychiatrist, and that this would have been less likely anywhere else. (4am27) My positive will be . . . that UCSF forced me to make a decision about what to do with my life, to take a year off, to solidify my ideas so as not to just go into something. It will also be that people were friendly and discussed things here, including faculty but especially residents and internists. (3wm24)

At the same time, UCSF students are disconcerted by the school's sheer intensity, compounded, they say, by the fact that the university offers only health-sciences degrees. They object that an innovative first biennium is followed by a more conventional one during which clinical faculty often appear too busy to teach, as at Minnesota, and high-tech more than primary-care medicine is extolled. One regrets that the students' diversity could be, but is not, mirrored among faculty.

- [The negative] for me is that the medical school at UCSF has no undergraduate campus associated with it. This plus the fact that it is in the city makes it more difficult to meet people with other interests than medicine. Most people in the city are working and it is very difficult to mix. Student life is less interesting since this is just a health-sciences campus. It lacks both intellectual and social diversity for this reason. (3wm24)
- For me [it] is that we put ourselves under such a high degree of stress. Medical school is stressful, the career is stressful. The question is, how could UCSF help this? I guess I do not know. I do know that at UCLA, medical students have a big sib[ling] program and must get together one or two times. Twenty-five percent participate in the program. (4am27) For me too, it is that there is so much to do . . . such a sense of responsibility . . . such a sense of "a lot." I do not feel that my time is my own. I find it hard to sleep and hard to wake up. Sometimes I have gotten more and more behind. I suppose it is more related to medicine than to UCSF. It is just tough to fully leave your work. Not

being a student for a while, for this reason, made it easier to come back to. Also, I did not like the lack of clarity of what you should learn in the clinical years. Everyone is so busy that it is not a good learning environment. It is a credit to the survival skills of students that they learn what they need to learn in these 2 years. The school can do much more, especially in the third-year transition period. (4wf31) I also think that fourth-year students are left too much to their own devices. (4wf31)

- What I do not like is that people evaluate you on the first week of your rotation when it takes 2 weeks to get a focus and even figure out what to do. (3wm24) I cannot think of a negative in the first 2 years except that I have been scared that I am not prepared for the third year. (2wf23) I feel that there is a kind of hypocrisy here. UCSF makes a point of choosing a diverse group, including socially. But then the role models are the big medical technicians and you have very little of the human element here. Teaching is rewarded in the preclinical years but not in the third and fourth years. Many of the clinicians who are doing primary-care work, for example, in teen pregnancy or drug abuse, are not recognized. There are also plenty of Chicanos, Asians, and blacks who are qualified and could teach well at UCSF. But there are very few of them on the faculty. (4hf30)

Students' views of what will be least beneficial in retrospect are also related to the school's unmitigated intensity and to its still-conventional curricular configuration.

- The negative will be that I gave up a lot. I sacrificed a lot to gain this education. I experienced a lot of delayed gratification. I am now 30 years old and would like to have three or four children by now. (4hf30) Although I may have been taught well, I will not have felt personally nurtured. At UCSF I have felt anonymous, in fact. It could, of course, be my own self-perception. I am very independent. I had some complaints about Yale in the same way. But I know that I am not the only one who feels as I do. (4wf31) Ditto, but I have found a couple of people to offset this with. (4hf30) I

will be in psychiatry 10 years from now and my wish will
be that I had learned more social sciences and interaction
stuff in medical school. (4am27) In 10 years I still will not
like how I was just dropped into the third year. I would do
the medicine and surgery rotations very differently now. I
would have liked to see more patients in the first and second years too. (3wm24)

McMaster pleasantly surprises its students, one by having
actually admitted him, others by having helped them dodge less
compelling careers, another by providing a conducive learning
environment. They like the school's trademark problem-based
small-group learning and integration of basic science and clinical instruction. They also enjoy the respect given them by clinicians, the curriculum's emphasis on communication skills, the
strong electives program, and the 3–year course of studies. Mc-
Master evokes loyalty to program and method.

- I was a science undergraduate at the University of Waterloo and was not thinking of medicine initially. After 3
  years at Waterloo, I applied to the MD program at McMaster and got in. I thought I would not get in but I was more
  drawn to McMaster than to any other medical school.
  (2wm22) My undergraduate degree in psychology and philosophy is from a small university in Ontario . . . where a
  large amount of learning takes place in small groups. I
  went to graduate school in psychology at Queens University in Kingston, Ontario, where I worked in the neurosur-
  gical unit. That is where . . . I discovered how much I dis-
  liked lecturing. It was very difficult to try to connect with
  180 kids three times a week in a lecture format. It was very
  difficult to make it work, both in terms of content and evaluation. Then, in the midst of work for the PhD, I interviewed for a place in the MD program here and was rejected 3 years running. The following year I applied and
  got in and the program allowed me to finish the PhD in the
  meantime. This is the only medical school that I could apply to because I do not have organic chemistry. [Here] I like
  the opportunity to work with people in small groups. I like
  the tutorial system at McMaster and the chance to learn

from fellow students. At McMaster I do not feel that my lack of a basic-science background limits me, and this is partly because of the tutorial system and the fact that we learn from each other here. The second thing I like about McMaster is the opportunity to work in groups outside the major tutorial groups, such as those in communication skills and clinical skills. I like very much the horizontal electives system at McMaster and the fact that in neuro-surgery already I have "cut skull." In this regard, I like very much the integration of clinical experience into the first couple of years in the MD program. (1wm26) The positives for me include the group learning environment, the fact that from the start students are treated with a lot of respect on the wards and tutorials and everywhere, and, the high point for me, the fact that one can pursue any elective whatsoever on an ongoing basis. In this regard I got the chance a year ago to help deliver a baby! I am still riding that wave. Imagine! I was in my second month of medical school! I graduated in 1991 from the University of Western Ontario with a major in genetics and an agricultural focus but in the fourth year I concluded that I could not improve upon the corn flake and thus became interested in genetics and medical research. I applied to Western Ontario, Queens, and McMaster, all in medicine. The varied background of students at McMaster was an advantage for me with respect to admission, compared to the other two universities, and I knew that I would have more control over my learning here. (2wm23)

- It is the problem-based learning format. Having done a fair amount of research before coming to McMaster, I think that problem-based learning fits right where I am. I also like the fact that the program takes only three years to complete and goes on continuously without a break. I like very much the integrated aspect of the program, the fact that it offers me much more clinical experience than any other medical school would. Here you read about certain elements, then you go into a practice setting and see them work. This really motivates you and drives you back and forth, from and to the books. (1wm28) [I: Do you ever have the sense of never finishing, given that there are no natural boundaries, no notes to memorize, no routine exams in the McMaster curriculum?] The type of closure that one gets in completing a chapter in a traditional learning format provides a false sense of security. In problem-based learning, when you fulfill your own objective, it provides a true sense of completion and is far better than a traditional exam. (2wm22) At McMaster, we feed off of not knowing that we are through. It is like admitting that you have to keep learning. The beauty of it is in the fact that we are lifetime learners. (2wm23) This is part of the belief system here. It is a system in which you realize how little you know, not how much you know, and in which you learn how to learn as an ongoing process. (1wm28) In the traditional system, the learner builds on the shoulders of others, whereas here at McMaster, learning instead resides in the belief of how little we actually know. At McMaster, you go from the ward back to the books. Is being unsure of how much you know, after all, a minus? I personally am more comfortable with the teaching that one knows less rather than that one knows this or that, period. (1wm26) [Tracing a snake-like up-and-down curve.] This represents the anxiety level in a traditional exam system, with anxiety plunging after the completion of an exam, then rising again toward the deadline for the next exam. This is the constant level of anxiety concerning how much one knows in a problem-based learning curriculum. I prefer the straight line over the precipitous rise and fall. (2wm23) The real strength of the system is that it is so different from the dissertation-writing process, where when you finish it, you just quit with it. (1wm26) This is all consistent with the noncompetitive atmosphere here at McMaster. (2wm22) The result of the ongoing and constant evaluation of students here is that every day you learn how well you performed that day. (1wm28)

But McMaster students also worry whether the recently introduced, and controversial, objective knowledge test or the possibility of extending the MD program to 4 years might not depart too much from "the way." All agree, however, though without mentioning lectures, that tutors might also be encouraged to teach.

- This school and this program . . . the consistency of student learning and excellence depends on the belief that the system will work. But it can break down. The tutorial system can break down when people do not have the goals of the system clearly in mind. I am one of the few students who is concerned about it, but many of us are looking for guidance. (1wm26) The negative here is in the student evaluation of tutors. The forms we must fill out are so redundant. They ask how tutors do this and how tutors do that and it all just leaves me wondering what on earth they want with all this information. I would prefer a much simpler evaluation, maybe five or six lines. (2wm22) My difficulty being in such an innovative program as McMaster is the difference between the training that I am receiving here and the content of qualifying exams that all students have to pass nationwide to be licensed. (1wm26) They recently designed a multiple-choice test to prepare us for the national exams. The goal is not so much to rank you in your class as to give you an indication of how you are progressing. (2wm23) But I am not sure that it measures learning or knowledge at all, and I am afraid that students will judge it this way, that they will judge the scores as a concrete index of their knowledge. I personally am against the test, but I also know that most students here are comfortable with multiple-choice exams and will not object. (1wm26)
- On the negative side is the fact that, with the 3–year program at McMaster and the clinical clerkship beginning in April, we have to make career choices before we even finish clinical rotations. I think this affects us and McMaster adversely. A lot of medical schools run the clerkships in the third year for this reason. (2wm23)
- The drawbacks of McMaster for me include a certain confusion generated by students' immersion in the formal language of the system. It is a language of issues, objectives, tutorials and so forth, virtually a foreign language compared to what you are actually learning. Also, I would like for there to be some teaching here! I know that at McMas-

ter we hate the word "teaching" or "teacher," but I personally would like more teaching about how to do things right.
I do not want teachers to tell us what to learn, but I do
want them at least to tell us that we are setting the objectives correctly that will help us learn. (1wm28) I actually
agree, and this gets back to my negative too, namely, how
the system depends on students' belief in it. (1wm26)

Sherbrooke wanted students and faculty alike to undertake the new pedagogy before passing judgment. So doing,
many have come to appreciate self-directed problem-based
learning as well as the new closeness to the clinical life of the
hospital and between teachers and students in general. Efforts
to better integrate basic science and clinical content in tutorials
are also praised. Sherbrooke is now attaching students to the
program as closely as McMaster long has.

- I like a lot of things at Sherbrooke. I can see now that I
  have progressed in a certain way of thinking. By last
  March I was very tired of tutorials, but when I arrived back
  in September I realized their importance to getting the scientific base in order to do the third-year multi-systems integration and clinical approach. Now I see the logic of the
  program. Another thing . . . is that from the start we are
  very close to the clinical life of the hospital . . . always in
  the hospital, always in contact with teachers and patients.
  It is very different from a program in which there are 200
  people in a lecture hall and one lecturer. Our teachers
  share a lot with us. The first year is less clinical, but in the
  second year already the doctors bring us to the patients.
  (3wf25) We learn to be very independent in our ways of doing things. We develop our own ways here at Sherbrooke. It
  really happens. (3wf24) For me it has been and still is the
  personal approach that I like the most. I am not in class
  with 150 kids. There is a lot of interaction both with doctors and students. I am actively participating in my studies. (3wm26) The principal advantage is the free time and
  the freedom of scheduling. (3wm31) The rewarding thing
  for me is the nonspoon-feeding methods learned at
  Sherbrooke. Like the New Pathway program at Harvard

shown recently on [the PBS (Public Broadcasting System) program] "NOVA," at Sherbrooke I can choose what is important for me. In a more traditional school, the first year would be set . . . just gross anatomy, histology, microbiology, biochemistry, and so forth. I like not having to do it this way. In the tutorial system, we integrate this content with living problems. In a traditional program I would be sitting in a class wondering what the importance is of metabolizing glucose. In tutorial, I ask what the importance is and we work on it within the context of a problem. It cuts out the excess and the superfluous in general. After all, we are not going to be specialists and researchers, most of us. (3wm25)

Sherbrooke students, like those at UCSF and Case Western Reserve, imagine appreciating in retrospect that the school encouraged them to remain whole persons and taught them with a human face how to learn in both self-directed and group-oriented ways.

- I imagine that I will continue having a life with an artistic side. I decided on medicine very late. I was never going to do just medicine. (3wf25) First, there is the learning aspect. I think that in 5 years I will see that I have learned how to learn, how to keep up-to-date, how to be an active learner. I will have had the experience of continuous learning. Second, there is the humanistic approach, and this is not a joke here. Even interacting in a small group has a humanistic effect. (3wm26) We learn to work in a group, in a team, and to adapt to our differences. (3wf25) The positive from the viewpoint 5 years hence will perhaps be the group dimension. (3wm31) The primary positive will be the experience at Sherbrooke as a whole, and particularly the self-directed learning method. I do not anticipate any labeling aspect to having attended Sherbrooke. Sherbrooke graduates are very popular in Moncton, New Brunswick. (3wm25)

But Sherbrooke students also think that too little basic-science knowledge is imparted, that tutorials are uneven in quality, and that a certain open-endedness or lack of structure is apparent in the new order, which leaves some not knowing what to expect compared to the old.

- Sometimes we do not do enough of the details. (3wf24) We should have students doing more anatomy in the first year, for instance, but it is not a problem exclusive to the new curriculum. (3wf25) But Sherbrooke was like this even before the reform, and not every student needs a body. You forget a lot of the details anyway. (3wm25) Even so I think there could be more controlled learning in anatomy. In each system, you could have a chance to dissect the organ. Some of the teachers are not quite clear concerning what their role is either. There is too much difference between one tutor and another. Some are better and some are worse. (3wf25) In the tutorial system, some people who are not interested in teaching have to teach nonetheless. (3wm25)
- Because our program is student oriented, you are left on your own pretty much. This is great, because you can learn yourself. Still, there is such a time constraint here. You are constantly asking the tutor what you should read before the next meeting and in the end there is still a test to take. I would like to spend more time on one subject or another, let's say, but then I find myself asking the tutor what I need to read for the exam. In a traditional program, you know what to expect. In this program, you are not sure what to expect. That has been the problem for me. (3wm26) It would be helpful to have some formal structure, not necessarily an exam, to guide students concerning what they have to know for the program . . . and they are working on it. (3wf25) We read and we read and we do not know what is pertinent. (3wm31) Yes, but you also learn to classify problems that way. (3wf24) To filter out the significant from the nonsignificant. (3wm25)

Finally, Sherbrooke students express a Quebecois "it will all work out" ethic, even as they anticipate, several years into their practices, recollecting irrelevant electives and rotations and a feeling of personal isolation at a medical center physically detached from the university itself.

- The big negative that I imagine is that the medical profession is not ready for an artist doctor, not to mention a woman surgeon. But this is a problem not really with the program at Sherbrooke but rather with the profession. The important thing is to adapt to this program, and certain kinds of personality do this very well. (3wf25) [I: Will there be any labeling effect in your medical practices from having attended Sherbrooke?] No. (All.) Anyway, I think that we will all learn in residency programs what we have not learned in the undergraduate program. (3wf25) The negative might be the system of electives and clinical rotations. In each case, the pertinence to actual medical training is questionable. Really, all you do is follow the doctors around. (3wm31) The only negative I can see is that for these 3 years at the faculty of medicine we have been separated from the University of Sherbrooke. We are on completely different campuses. There is a social aspect to this. It has nothing to do with the program per se, but I feel that I am stuck with my hundred colleagues here. I feel that I am segregated and isolated with the medical students. There may be 60–some girls of 100 in every medical school class here, but I would like to be closer to the university as a whole. I think it really retards social life being here. (3wm25)

Conclusion

What have we learned about innovation in general professional medical education in the course of this study? To begin with, we have found that change as we define it is a process in parts, each part a partial answer to the question, "Why?" By method and intent, therefore, our method is Aristotelian, in searching out the material, formal, efficient, and telic determinants of change.[1]

The underlying assumption, which distinguishes this work from more "targeted" policy studies, is that while innovation content is quite variable over time, innovation process is rather constant. Even restricting the locus of change examined to teaching and learning practice, as we have, it is clear that the "family" of innovative ideas from which each of our 10 schools has selected over the present reform cycle—ideas inscribed in the several dozen recommendations of the 1984 *GPEP Report* presented in Appendix 2—is a highly extended one. We have not wanted to fix inquiry upon any particular family member, therefore, first, because there are so many such; second, because local circumstances affect how any one is configured and applied on-site; and, third, because each application is itself so soon adjusted as inside evidence, and new program evaluation mounts and outside shifts occur in educational and societal preferences.

It seemed to us more useful to ascertain the relatively content-independent mechanics of innovation process per se, whether that process may have unfolded in the 1970s, 1980s, or 1990s. In this, we drew from David Riesman's notion that the "academic procession," viewed from above and in the aggregate, is not linear but snake-like, such that, at any one moment, the head can take an innovative turn that may require considerable time to register back through the coils. No one segment in other words, no one school or band of schools, is ever found to be moving in the exactly same direction as another segment at any one time over the course of a reform cycle, though each may imagine itself, from its perspective, very much in tune with the times (Riesman, 1961). The point is nicely illustrated in one respondent's account of how the MD program at McMaster University, at the very head of the medical education innovation procession through the 1970s and '80s, may be taking just such a turn in the mid-1990s.

- I was hired [originally] to do research on problem-solving skills. I was concerned to find measures of these skills. Now I realize that you cannot do this until you have specified content. We now know, in other words, that the search for problem-solving skills in the absence of content is a search for the Holy Grail. I do not look at problem-solving skills anymore because it is not a useful construct. In my view, it was a rhetorical ploy that captures the flavor of that time. [I: What is wrong with the construct?] Skills devoid of knowledge are meaningless. [I: Then what purpose did the construct of problem-based learning serve?] Mobilization. The enemy was the traditional medical school, and the idea that the more knowledge you transmit the more learning takes place. This notion is still dead wrong, and problem-based learning was in fact a step forward in dissociating learning from teaching. Problem-based learning succeeded in disillusioning the traditional medical curriculum. Problem-based learning, for example, left students free time. [I: Then do you believe there is a third way, a synthesis?] Yes, I do. It is problem-based learning in the weak sense of the term, problem-based learning that plays a role in students apprehending content, in learning actively, in retaining knowledge, period. But in the strong sense, the sense in which problem-based learning is knowledge-free, problem-based learning is meaningless. We may say this quite clearly now in the 1990s and act upon it at McMaster, whereas in the 1960s and 1970s, if we had said it, we would never have gotten started. There would have been no motivation, and we would have lost the program. Over the years, as it happens, we oversold the change at McMaster by far. At present, we hold very few illusions and we are the true converts now.

FINDINGS

We have found noteworthy differences among schools in who and what prompts innovation, in how it is conceived, and in how it is effected and received. We have related these differences to the schools' missions (comprehensive or distinct), perceived problems (structural or situational), and attitudes of faculty (attached or detached), as well as to whether the schools are bigger or smaller, public or private, older or younger, and earlier or later innovators. We summarize here some of our main impressions from the experiences of these 10 schools and offer a few suggestions to other medical educators who may wish to learn from them.

The context of change—institutional mission and problems, school size and resources, and faculty morale—affects the nature and scope of the innovation that medical schools attempt.

More mission-distinct schools like Mercer, New Mexico, Hawaii, and the Canadians McMaster and Sherbrooke, more readily undertake MD-program-wide changeovers than more mission-comprehensive schools like Minnesota, Case Western Reserve, Dartmouth, Harvard, and the University of California, San Francisco [UCSF]. A more distinct mission—say, to prepare community-oriented physicians for generalist practices in a state or province—is associated in turn, we have observed, with more of a "captain" than "referee" style of leadership and, not surprisingly, is found more in the smaller, more compact schools than in the larger, more far-flung.

A more comprehensive mission—to train for specialty practices and academic medicine, to conduct research at the most advanced levels, to staff tertiary-care academic health centers—may be sustained only by the larger do-it-all schools typically led by administrator deans. As referees among their schools' many interested contenders, these deans do well to captain any curricular project at all, let alone one in innovative teaching and learning practice. Spending on education, pre- and postdoctoral combined, rarely takes up more than a tenth of the budget at these schools, in any case.

If more distinct mission is associated with smaller schools and more comprehensive mission with larger, and if size in turn favors different styles of leadership, then we would expect change, in sponsorship and scope, to vary accordingly. We would expect it to be more top-down, administrator-led, and of broader scope at the former, more bottom-up, faculty-driven, and narrower in scope at the latter schools. And, indeed, this is what we do find, contrasting Mercer, Hawaii, and Sherbrooke, for example, with Minnesota, Case Western Reserve, and UCSF. This is not to say that a dean may not captain broader change at a big, mission-comprehensive school like Harvard, nor referee contending tracks at a smaller, mission-distinct school like New Mexico. It is only to report the central tendency. The dismay that we found at McMaster—no longer such a small program, given the growth that occurred over the 1980s—concerning the loss of community and institutional agility in the MD program is indicative of this tendency.

Bigger schools, like airplanes, fly less affected by turbulence than do smaller, more compact schools because they are heavier and can bring more equipment to bear. Minnesota's problems with the state's increasingly competitive health care environment, UCSF's with its spacial limits to growth, Case Western Reserve's with rising up the ranks of research schools, Harvard's with schoolwide funding limitations and rifts among reform currents, even smaller Dartmouth's with integrating the biomedical and clinical parts of its new academic health complex, are, for all their urgency, situational, not structural, in nature. They are at most medium-term problems and have identifiable solutions that, when implemented, promise improvement. Sherbrooke in contrast, and also Mercer in its first decade, illustrate how vulnerable the smallest and youngest medical school in a province or state may be when the entire region's political economy tumbles and education systems retrench. Here, solutions have had to match problems in scope. Thus at Sherbrooke, against threat of closure, a central administration transformed the entire curriculum, while at Mercer, in the upstart's struggle to survive, the ranking administration insists on keeping graduates mission-compliant in providing primary care to the state's underserved populations.

Morale, the greater or lesser identification of individuals with the whole school and its fortunes, as we have defined it, is also mission, associated with school size. Smaller schools like Mercer, Hawaii, New Mexico, and Sherbrooke can be institutionally abuzz in ways that bigger schools like Minnesota and UCSF cannot be. When a buzz develops over more structural problems—a dire financial setback or even a threat to survival—nearly everyone at the smaller schools can and does get involved for or against proposed solutions. At the bigger, more far-flung schools, where loyalties, hence morale, attach to discipline-based departments, even to subdepartment units, and where individuals can spend whole careers wholly engaged in medical research and advanced practice, only the exceptional dean as at Harvard or UCSF, and then only for limited time periods, can focus faculty attention on any one program- or schoolwide issue.

As favored as the smaller, more compact schools may be in more readily initiating and designing broad change than their bigger, more complex counterparts, they may be less favored in implementing and institutionalizing changeovers. Thus, we have found that the administrator-led transformations of curriculum designed at smaller schools like Hawaii, New Mexico, and Sherbrooke can face greater uncertainty with respect to lasting effects, than the more bounded faculty- or faculty–administrator-sponsored adjustments effected recently at Minnesota, UCSF, Dartmouth, and McMaster. Faculty at the former can feel displaced from primary discipline–department affiliation and overwhelmed by the pace and demands of change. Second-generation innovators at these schools face the "disciples' dilemma," moreover, or how to institutionalize the charisma that first gave impetus and concept to big change. Innovation brought top-down is more easily swept away in active or passive resistance by the rank and file than more modest efforts built bottom-up, more experimentally, by faculty or faculty–administrator combinations.

Schools' defining characteristics—their public-private,

older-younger, and earlier-later innovator status—have also been found to affect the nature and scope of innovation. First, and counter to expectation, we observed that in aggregate the public schools, those tied juridically and fiscally to state legislatures, innovate schools. Granted that the study's more global innovators, Hawaii, New Mexico, Sherbrooke, and (one-third state-supported) Mercer are not only public but also smaller medical schools, and that the more modest approaches observed at Minnesota and UCSF suggest a size effect, being public appears at least not to have hindered broad change efforts at four of six such schools. There is little evidence here, therefore, holding leadership constant, that the greater autonomy of private institutions prompts bolder experiments. It may be that eventual accountability to a state legislature actually quickens the adaptive response in some instances. Second, though the older schools are disproportionately the larger ones, we found that the younger schools in this study, those founded during or after the expansive 1960s by our definition, are, including the two Canadians, the broader-scope curriculum innovators. In this there is some hint of a cohort- and/or age-induced propensity to greater risk-taking. Third, we have heard enough at earlier innovators Case Western Reserve, Minnesota, and McMaster—in testimony concerning how well present-day discipline-departmental and research-clinic revenue imperatives efface collective memory of past reform practice—to credit the notion that "having innovated profoundly" might in time dampen the impulse to "innovate profoundly again" under new circumstances.

Though the older schools are also disproportionately the larger, it is also suggestive that the younger schools, those founded after 1960 by our definition, are, including the two Canadians, the broader-scope curriculum innovators of the study. Perhaps this is a consequence of a convergence of the goals of reform and the founding rationales for the newer schools.

As for the students, we found few differences among schools—despite variations in mission, problems, and morale as well as juridical, age, and innovator status—in what students most appreciate. They invariably value those parts of their instruction that encourage individuation and independent learning, on the one hand, and connection, to students, faculty, patients, and communities, on the other. They also always prize diversity, in the various ways that it may be manifested in their midst.

Differences do emerge in what students least appreciate, however. At Mercer, Hawaii, New Mexico, Sherbrooke, and Mc-Master especially, smaller, mission-distinct schools where various present-reform-cycle-options—small-group, problem-based, student-centered, basic–clinical science integrated, patient- and community-oriented medical instruction—have been broadly implemented, students dislike those parts of their programs that provide too much new pedagogy and too little standard instruction. Conversely, at Minnesota, Case Western Reserve, Harvard, UCSF, and Dartmouth, larger (save the latter), mission-comprehensive schools where the same new options have been more narrowly or selectively implemented within more or less conventional curricula, students tend to dislike the parts of their programs that provide too much standard instruction and too little new pedagogy.

Dramatic advances in biomedical research over the past half century have dramatically reshaped the medical schools as faculties have grown to include ever larger numbers of increasingly specialized researchers and clinicians preoccupied with the search for renewed support from government, industry, and practice plans. Valuable and necessary as these actors have been in advancing cutting-edge research and technically current clinical care, their organization into discipline-based departments and related subunits has reinforced narrow professionalism, restricted intellectual vistas, and undermined the teaching role. Not surprisingly therefore, at the schools that we have studied, department interests and the research- and clinic-revenue imperative are consistently portrayed as obstacles to reform in general professional medical education. If the determined deans and reform-minded faculty that we have met have countered successfully with a variety of organizational strategies, incentives, and persuasion, it is also telling how rarely their efforts reach beyond biomedical sciences instruction to include the clinical phase of pre- and postdoctoral medical education. This, in our view, along with the emerging links among molecular, patient-centered, and population-based models of physician education, represents the next frontier in physician instruction.

SUGGESTIONS

What may these findings suggest to the broader community of medical educators?

From the students, whose testimony was reported in part 3, come two suggestions. First, more traditional lecture-lab programs contemplating innovation of the sorts we have studied should trust that well-considered efforts of any scope to introduce small-group, problem-based, independent, integrated teaching and learning will be deeply appreciated by most students. The greater the effort, we found, the more enthusiastic the students. Second, programs that would make broad change-overs, transformations of entire curricula or entire rows or columns of curricula, should note that, at schools too hastily reconfigured in these ways, students, aware that they must soon compete in the unreconfigured postdoctoral world, want effective instruction per se. The more effective their instruction—lecture, lab, or tutorial—the more enthusiastic the students. Less well-considered changeovers can leave whole-class cohorts resentful and uncertain.

From the educators, whose testimony was reported in parts 1 and 2, come two suggestions as well. First, if you are an MD program in a bigger, more mission-comprehensive, department–discipline-based medical school within a more complex academic medical center, and your goal is to reconfigure general professional medical education selecting from a variety of current-reform-cycle options, understand that faculty- or faculty-administrator-sponsored within-bounds efforts gradually implemented in more specific areas[2] may go with the institutional grain better than more general curricular conversions; such specific curricular adjustments, however, may produce so little aggregate change in educational practice as to leave many faculty and students unaffected, thus maintaining the status quo.

If, on the other hand, you are an MD program in a smaller, more mission-distinct, less department–discipline-based medical school within a less complex academic medical center, and your goal is to reconfigure likewise, understand that administrator- or administrator–faculty-sponsored across-the-board efforts swiftly implemented in more general areas[3] may go with the institutional grain better than more specific curricular adjustments; such general curricular conversions, however, may produce so much aggregate change in educational practice as to leave many faculty and students overwhelmed, thus inviting regression to the status quo.

Schools interested in changing general professional medical education practice are advised, then, to know themselves sufficiently well to choose wisely among possible ends-in-view and rationally among suitable means to these ends. We have reported the experience of ten successful innovators, and drawn inferences from their efforts, not because we think that these findings may simply be reproduced at other sites, but because a method to change may be revealed. Always, change effort of any scope begins with impetus and insight, and proceeds, in the presence of opportunity and sponsorship, through design to implementation. Consequences, intended and unintended, provide the data for subsequent elaborations. We hope that somewhere in the process that we have detailed, useful information may be gleaned for the next series of iterations.

NOTES

1. Proposed to explain the development of phenomena in nature (*physikê*, acorn-to-oak, for example). Aristotle's four causes—"four meanings of the question 'why' [including] the material out of which an object is generated . . . the form (*eidos*) or pattern (*paradeigma*) . . . the [efficient or] immediate source of change [or] 'determining agency' (*aitia*) . . . the end (*telos*) or purpose for the sake of which a thing is done"—parallel the parts of our own effort to explain the development of an institution in society (*politikê*) in both intent and method (full accounting of a complex, step-wise, cumulating process over time). Thus our impetus (innovators' will, organized efforts) would correspond to Aristotle's material causation, our design (thinking through alternatives) to his formal causation, our implementation (putting concept into practice) to his efficient causation, our mission (putting vision into concept) to his telic causation. See the selections from sections ii ("The province of natural science," pp. 24–25), iii ("The four types of explanation," pp. 25–29), and vii ("Relations of the four determining factors, pp. 35–37) in Book II ("The Conditions of Natural Occurrences") of *Natural Science* in Philip Wheelwright, Ed., trans., *Aristotle* (pp. 26 and 35 for the preceding quotation).

2. For example, more basic sciences–clinical correlations (as at Minnesota), small-group tutorial additions to lecture courses (UCSF), early clinic ex-

posure to patients (Case Western Reserve), ambulatory care clerkships (Dartmouth), a separate society for experimental curricula (Harvard), "burden of illness" epidemiological course content (McMaster).

3. Small-group problem-based learning in replacement of lecture–lab instruction (variously at Mercer, Hawaii, Sherbrooke), mission-mandated primary-care specialization (Mercer), community-based clerkships (Hawaii), primary-care and traditional-curriculum track merging (New Mexico), extension of problem-based learning into third- and fourth-year clinical "mentorial" instruction (Sherbrooke).

Voices for Change

If the 1980s began on an upbeat, with a major reassessment of the structure and function of undergraduate medical education expressed in the *GPEP Report* (Muller, 1984), the decade ended on a downbeat, with broad dismay about how little had changed, and even greater urgency in calls for change. Here, we review five of the most cogent of these calls—those of Robert Ebert and Eli Ginzberg, David Greer, Charles Odegaard, Kerr White, and the Pew Health Professions Commission—among the many that were being voiced by the early 1990s. Our effort will be to weave their separate analyses into a comprehensive commentary ordered in five sections, as follows: societal forces (social, demographic, scientific); school structure (paradigm, mission, curriculum); internal authority (leadership, governance, faculty); external authorities (major payers, discipline and profession, licensing and accreditation); and school functions (instruction, research, selection and admission). The first paragraph of each subsection summarizes the problem.

Societal Forces

Social

A profound shift is underway in people's attitudes toward the medical profession. Manifestations of the change are said to include patients' and families' mounting insistence on a more active role in medical decisions, the recent avalanche of malprac-

Adapted from *Health Affairs,* Volume 7:2, Supplement 1981, pp. 5–38. "The Reform of Medical Education," by Ebert and Ginzberg. The People-to-People Health Foundation, Inc. Project HOPE. All rights reserved.

tice litigation, deep concern by the public and by their politicians over mounting medical costs, and a broad redefining of medicine's task to take account of the perceived needs and attributes of the individuals and populations served.

Health professions education is "out of step with the evolving health needs of the American people," Thomas Langfitt declares, introducing the Pew Commission's (1991) report (p. iii). Countless "micro-systems," which constitute the present health care delivery system, are working badly today.

> The ordering of diagnostic tests is incoherent and excessive. Medical and surgical interventions are performed without a clear understanding of the expected outcomes by either the physicians or the patients. Social and emotional factors that contribute to the patients' illnesses are lost in the rush. Little attention is given to strategies that will help prevent recurrence of those particular illnesses . . . [a]nd many incurable patients are not allowed to die at their request and with dignity. (Pew, 1991, p. iv)

If the root problem is at the microsystem level, which "no amount of restructuring or refinancing at the macro level will correct," then change, Langfitt concludes, "must begin with a new vision of what health professionals ought to be doing that they are not doing today. In general terms, they need to be closer to the patients and their families . . . to understand better why people behave the way they do, particularly under stress" (Pew, 1991, p. iv).

On the demand side, the Pew Commission (1991, p. 8) foresees mounting consumer empowerment due to "shifting expectations, an emphasis on health promotion and growing consumer cost sharing." Issues including "informed consent, litigiousness, quality assurance and cost containment" will become more dramatic in the years ahead. Information will further demystify medicine and personal health for the better educated and heighten expectations concerning wellness in the later years. Consumers will be actively involved in health maintenance, wellness, exercise, and dietary programs, in self-diagnosis and treatment technologies, and even in medical decisions, and they will expect greater accountability, effectiveness, and efficiency. Cost control, the Commission writes, will also be a determinant:

[C]oordinated care will become more prevalent as financial pressures increase [prompting expansion] from a system focused solely on the provision of individual care to a system that also addresses overall population health . . . diversification in the mix of providers . . . alteration in who delivers care to whom, when and where . . . lower-cost settings . . . ambulatory and community-based alternatives to . . . hospitalization . . . mechanisms to continually and systematically measure outcomes . . . encourage practitioner accountability and standardize patterns of practice. (Pew, 1991, p. 6)

Reporting impressions of a 1987 conference, "The Task of Medicine," Kerr White notes participants' sense of "massive societal discontent and discordance between medicine's and society's perceptions of the task" (White, 1988, p. 13). Attitude change of this magnitude is "at the root of the revolution in which medicine now finds itself—a revolution precipitated in part by the molecular and technological revolutions wrought by biomedicine and in part by our widespread failure to assimilate large amounts of extra-somatic or non-biological experience and information" (p. 30). Consequently, White too sees a shift in viewpoint, from "a 'supply' dominated model of medicine's task, controlled by the country's medical schools, to a 'demand' dominated model based on the perceived needs and attributes of the individuals and populations served" (p. 31). Even so, he observes, "many segments of the American public share a widely held belief that every problem has a solution, that every solution involves a pill, procedure or some other intervention or service, and that every service has . . . a 'provider!' " (p. 67).

On the supply side, David Greer worries, the medical profession's inadequate response to mounting social dissatisfaction has engendered a host of "unorthodox practitioners, paramedical professionals, healers, and technicians of a wide variety of persuasions [who] have experienced growing social acceptance in recent years and . . . increased their efforts to move the medical profession aside to make room for their more limited and frequently less scientific approaches to health care" (Greer, 1990, p. 212).

Demographic

By century's end the U.S. will have twice the number of physicians per 1,000 population that it had at mid-century. At the same time, managed care systems will use fewer physicians than fee-for-service practices have generally used and specialists will be less in demand because of the constraints to referral that managed care health delivery systems impose. Demand for physicians' services may drop significantly, therefore, quantitatively and qualitatively.

Reviewing projections, Robert Ebert and Eli Ginzberg put the average number of physicians per 100,000 population presently at between 220 and 230 for the U.S., up from 140 just after World War II (Ebert & Ginzberg, 1988). By the turn of the century, they predict, it will stand at 270 to 280. Compounding the oversupply problem will be the large number of foreign medical graduates (FMGs) who have entered the country since the 1960s—Asians and Latin Americans, but also U.S citizens graduated from Mexican, Caribbean, and European medical schools—recruited to fill residency positions in the community and public hospitals.

At the same time, Ebert and Ginzberg suggest, growth of prepaid plans will reduce demand for physicians inasmuch as such plans, which deliver care to designated groups, employ only about 100 physicians per 100,000, about half the national ratio. Physician surplus will be greater, therefore, in proportion to the growth of these plans. Parallel growth of managed-care plans foreshadows decline in referrals to specialists, inasmuch as these patients, unlike those in fee-for-service arrangements, are not free to consult specialists as they wish (Ebert & Ginzberg, 1988).

Scientific

Molecular biology now pervades the frontiers of many biomedical sciences, and these sciences are increasingly distanced from patients' bedside. Medical educators are often left wondering which aspects of contemporary biological science are most pertinent to the actual practice of medicine. Some now question the validity of emphasizing the most current work in biological science in teaching medical students.

Three decades' development of biomedical science and technology, in the Pew Commission's view, has led to "amazing growth" in diagnostic and therapeutic capabilities.

The growth of biotechnology, such as genetically based diagnostic and treatment capabilities, will redefine the meaning of illness, disease prevention, health and health care. . . . The effects of biotechnology will continue to unfold over the entire practice life of today's health professional students, and they will be challenged to anticipate the transition and lead the way in interpreting clinical practice within its context. (Pew, 1991, pp. 7–8)

Advances in knowledge and technique in molecular biology "have progressed at a pace that surprises even those who work in this field," the Pew Commission (1991, p. 47) remarks, a pace that "makes possible a range of research, diagnostic and treatment methods undreamed of just a few decades ago." Examples include mapping the entire human genome, recombinant deoxyribonucleic acid (DNA) technology, genetic probes and markers, and gene replacement therapy. Yet the growing volume and rising rate of change of biomedical information, the Commission concludes, also poses a direct educational challenge. Physician education must become "more efficient in effectively training professionals and must also endow them with a lifelong curiosity and desire to learn" (1991, pp. 48–49). Of great promise in this regard are developments, for example, in medical informatics that link a student's personal computer software, cardiac monitor, and human torso replica in order to teach critical-care medicine; and of teaching modules that use high-resolution visual images to integrate organ-specific material from gross anatomy, histology, pathology, radiology, physiology, and biochemistry in a problem-solving, interactive learning environment.

School Structure

Paradigm

In 1910 Flexner wrote that though the "fundamental sciences . . . furnish the essential instrumental basis of medical education" that base "can hardly serve as the permanent professional minimum." Rather, practitioners must deal with "facts of two categories." If the former were imparted by physics, chemistry, and biology, Flexner continued, the latter require a "different apperceptive and appreciative apparatus" insofar as physicians' work "is fast becoming social and preventive, rather than individual and curative" (Flexner, 1910, p. 26). Yet fully eight decades later Flexner's broader paradigm is still to be widely accepted.

The following passage from *The Flexner Report,* Odegaard writes, might interest medical educators who still consider the "Flexnerian" curriculum—firm scientific bases followed by practical clinical experience within a university research setting—orthodoxy.

> [T]he fundamental sciences . . . furnish the essential instrumental basis of medical education. But the instrumental minimum can hardly serve as the permanent professional minimum. It is even instrumentally inadequate. The practitioner deals with facts of two categories. Chemistry, physics, biology enable him to apprehend one set; he needs a different apperceptive and appreciative apparatus to deal with the other, more subtle elements. Specific preparation is in this direction much more difficult; one must rely for the requisite insight and sympathy on a varied and enlarging cultural experience. Such enlargement of the physician's horizon is otherwise important, for scientific progress has greatly modified his ethical responsibility. His relation was formerly to his patient—at most to his patient's family; and it was almost always remedial. The patient had something the matter with him; the doctor was called in to cure it. Payment of a fee ended the transaction. But the physician's function is fast becoming social and preventive, rather than individual and curative. Upon him society relies to ascertain, and through measures essentially educational to enforce, the conditions that prevent disease and make positively for physical and moral well-being. It goes without saying that this type of doctor is first of all an educated man. (Flexner, 1910, p. 26; Odegaard, 1986, pp. 12–14)

But first Flexner, then medical education, dropped the second set of facts, Odegaard regrets. Even in the *GPEP Report,* he finds a

> paucity of references . . . to the subject matter of the medical curriculum[, possibly] the result of deliberate intent on the part of its sponsor, the Association of American Medical Colleges. . . .

Despite the [Panel's] concern 'with defining the essential knowledge and fundamental skills' physicians should possess, there is no presentation in the report of essential knowledge, apart from the reference to the bench-mark Flexnerian curriculum. The invitation to 'debate on the personal qualities, values, and attitudes' appropriate for a physician does not lead to any references to subject matter and certainly not to any specific literature on the subject. (Odegaard, 1986, pp. 63–64)

Those who would now broaden the established curriculum will confront the many who still share the narrow biomedical view, notwithstanding a few broader formulations, Odegaard notes, such as Holly Smith's that the

boundaries of medicine blend into psychology, sociology, economics, and even into cultural heritage. Disease may be encoded in the genome; disease may also be encoded by the deprivations of poverty and ignorance. Medicine must therefore be concerned not only with an abnormal molecule but also with an abnormal childhood. . . . The practice of medicine is far more than the application of scientific principles to a particular biologic aberration. . . . [It] is tragically easy for the patient to become merely the repository in which a disease or a syndrome has chosen to manifest its[elf]. . . . Patients want to be listened to and understood . . . want physicians to be interested in them as fellow human beings . . . expect competence in medical science and technology . . . want to be kept reasonably informed . . . want not to be abandoned. [Though] the basic sciences . . . taught in medical schools . . . have reasonably defined margins . . . clinical medicine [is] an open-ended system of bewildering complexity in which science is blurred by sociology, psychology interacts with economics, traditions and ethical concepts are buffeted by new imperatives. (Smith, 1985; Odegaard, 1986, pp. 32–34)

In Alvin Tarlov's view, given in the preface to Kerr White's conference report (White, 1988, p. ix), the prevailing paradigm defines disease in terms of "disordered molecular and biochemical processes that engender cellular, tissue, organ, and system disturbance or destruction." Disease is thus a "characteristic constellation of specific biochemical, physiological, and pathological anomalies responsible for specific loss of physical and other functions experienced by the patient and observed by the physician."* Not surprisingly therefore, dissatisfaction with the prevailing paradigm has arisen and a broader one emerged, in part out of awareness that the same illness in patients' experience "may be as highly individualized as fingerprints" (Tarlov, cited in White, 1988, p. ix). Intended to broaden, not to replace, the prevailing view, Tarlov continues, the broader paradigm opens from biomedical to psychosocial, cultural, and economic factors to explain disease. In Tarlov's words,

> A broad range of social, cultural and economic factors . . . influence the state of health of individuals and nations. These influences include education, income level, racial and class status in society, customs and habits, advertising and other commercial practices, and the laws and regulations by which we are governed. These external factors, we now know, can have influences at any point or on many points along the chain of events in the prevailing paradigm: biochemical, cellular and system function; disease onset and course; individual illness response; level of functioning in everyday activities; psychological state; and response to therapy. Knowledge of these external factors and their effects on individual health should be incorporated into a revised intellectual foundation for medicine. (White, 1988, p. x)

Academic medicine's narrow view of health and disease, White charges, results from a profession's ignorance of its own history, and of the history of science and the humanities in general, and, consequently, its narrow definition of the boundaries and characteristics of science. It is ignorance that runs in the face of a "whole host of problems bearing on health and disease [that] cry out for . . . scientific enlightenment including evolution, morphogenesis, behavior, memory, personality, suffering, and caring" (White, 1988, pp. 9, 11). The definition is further restricted by the profession's equation of science and technology,

---

*White notes Donald Seldin's clear statement of the dominant perspective in most American medical schools: "Medicine is a very narrow discipline. Its goals may be defined as the relief of pain, the prevention of disability, and the postponement of death by the application of the theoretical knowledge incorporated in medical science to individual patients" (Seldin, 1981, p. 4).

the idea that the development and deployment of technology actually constitutes science. White says,

> To put it more bluntly, the emphasis in much narrowly defined biomedical research, particularly in clinical departments in recent decades, has been on "know how," rather than on "know why," "know whether," and "know what." . . . In too many teaching environments, concern with improving skills in instrumentation appears to take precedence over efforts to expand the information base for clinical understanding and reasoning, and for patient counseling and management. (White, 1988, p. 12)

Conference participants, White continues, clearly saw how the profession "sequesters" the very knowledge that an expanded model of health and illness makes available to it. For one example, patients' views of their problems and of the relationship of these to their life circumstances, are largely ignored, inasmuch as input of the sort cannot be measured or counted, but only experienced, reported, and observed. Academic medicine deals with molecules, cells, and organs far more easily than with people, individually and collectively. For another, the natural sciences have been so successful as to obscure other medically relevant disciplines in the schools. Many at the conference imagined

> broader and more inclusive ways of looking at individual and collective problems of health and disease. . . .. What is needed, first and foremost throughout academic medicine . . . is more, not less, and broader, not narrower, scientific thinking and scholarship . . . more and different types of . . . interaction with those sciences that Flexner's disciples excluded . . . psychology, anthropology, sociology, demography, economics, epidemiology, health statistics. (White, 1988, p. 19)

If Flexner (cited in Pew, 1991, p. 12) envisioned an educational arrangement "that helped us get out of an ill-fitting box" at the close of the last century, the Pew Commission likewise urges, so a new arrangement may now be envisioned that serves the same function in the present impasse, one that employs

> a richer array of academic disciplines, a more interactive relationship with the community and public, a more integrated con-

nection to the practice side of the profession, a greater openness to education and work across the health professions and a greater willingness to experiment with alternative structures for organizing the work of education, research and patient care. (Pew, 1991, pp. 11–12)

Mission

As evidence mounts that more primary-care physicians are needed, medical schools are being urged to re-orient students from specialty to primary care and to shift training and services from hospital wards to ambulatory settings. Pilot projects for patient care, education, and research might be set up in HMOs (health maintenance organizations), outreach clinics, and group practices, it is suggested, and faculty employed there to train medical students and residents. Inner-city and rural health centers might likewise be enlisted as learning labs in health maintenance, disease prevention, and clinical epidemiology.

Without a particular sense of mission, the Pew Commission (1991, p. 12) declares, "organizations do not know precisely which of literally thousands of opportunities that exist in the environment should be pursued." Mission is an organization's self-understanding in a world of competitors. "Without clear and distinctive statements of institutional mission, health professional schools will find it difficult to bring about long term change. Clarity of mission helps provide the vision for [creating] new types of schools and directs the full force of institutional resources to address those concerns" (Pew, 1991, p. 12).

Above all, mission must strike a balance between primary and tertiary care, Kerr White proposes.

Common problems are common and rare problems are rare! In the United States the overall system is grossly out of balance. The ratios of tertiary care beds and of many sub-specialists to ambulatory care facilities and to general physicians are reversed from those in most other industrialized countries. Appropriately trained primary care physicians are in short supply in the United States [in contrast to] Canada, Australia or New

Zealand. . . . [A] substantial part of almost two generations of leaders in American academic medicine . . . do[es] not understand what primary care is. . . . [F]ar too many members of the contemporary medical establishment, in both basic and clinical departments, do not seem to appreciate the challenges and opportunities for research in primary care. (White, 1988, p. 53)

An independent body such as the 1966 Millis Commission on Graduate Medical Education, White suggests, should now examine the question "whether primary care is just an 'add-on' to the real business of medicine, designed in effect to keep state legislators and consumer groups quiet, or whether American medical schools should assume collective responsibility for educating and training a primary care sector capable of looking after ninety percent of the population's health problems" (White, 1988, p. 73).

That body, White specifies, unlike the Millis Commission, which examined problems top-down from the teachers' and profession's perspective, should use a bottom-up population-based approach informed by data from the National Household Interview Survey, the National Ambulatory Medical Care Survey, the National Hospital Discharge Survey, and the Ambulatory Sentinel Practice Network, as well as from some of the larger HMOs and from health statistical sources in Britain, Canada, and other countries that were not available to the Millis Commission. Questions should concern the content of primary-care practice as defined by patients and the type of problems brought to this source of care and their distribution; the types of people who enjoy this kind of practice and do it well, their personality characteristics and aptitudes; whether making an appropriately trained cadre of "general physicians" (internists, family physicians, pediatricians) the majority of all physicians would reduce costs and improve the care of patients; which undergraduate and graduate education best transmits and sustains broad knowledge and skills needed by primary-care physicians; how research in primary-care questions can best be stimulated; what changes in resource allocation are necessary to achieve such goals.

Robert Ebert and Eli Ginzberg concur, urging that a majority of graduates should now be prepared to provide primary care without further training, that a small percentage should complete training in one or another of the specialties of medicine, and that an even smaller percentage should continue to train for academic medical research and teaching (Ebert & Ginzberg, 1988).

David Greer, too, challenges the major medical associations, specialty boards, and residency review committees to become more responsive to the needs of the general public.

> The need is for a 180–degree turn in educational perspective from the current [bioscientific] model . . . to a model that presents medicine to students as primarily a human service endeavor emerging from social need. . . . Students must be made to realize early in their education that medicine, despite its vigorous and laudatory attempts to expand its scientific foundation, is not a science; neither its orientation nor its methods, much less its goals, are those of the scientist. Medicine is a social service, a response to perceived communal as well as individual need, and should be so represented in medical education. (Greer, 1990, p. 220)

If, as they do, the professional schools depend on the support of the communities that they serve, Greer argues, the schools should pursue the needs and expectations of the latter. Medical educators in particular must understand that the majority of U.S. medical schools are public institutions and that even the privately sponsored institutions are largely supported by public sources. They must appreciate that over half the resources expended by U.S. academic medical centers come from public funds, by way of subsidies for patient care, tax deferrals, and grants and contracts.

Having always practiced fee-for-service medicine and made a living treating the financially capable part of the population, Greer charges, American physicians have never affirmed the public mission of medicine that Flexner and the Carnegie Foundation advocated early in the century and that E. A. Winslow, Yale Professor of Public Health, defined in 1920 as

> the science and art of preventing disease, prolonging life, and promoting physical health and efficiency through organized community efforts for the sanitation of the environment, the control of

community infections, the education of individuals in principles of personal hygiene, the organization of medical and nursing service for the early diagnosis and preventive treatment of disease, and the development of the social machinery which will ensure to every individual in the community a standard of living adequate for the maintenance of health. (Greer, quoting Winslow, 1990, pp. 206–207; Winslow, 1920, p. 30)

To the contrary, Greer regrets, the medical profession has actually considered the public mission radical, socialist, un-American, or "merely coddling [of] the unworthy who are not capable or willing to care for themselves" (Greer, 1990, p. 207). Nineteenth-century public dispensaries for treating the sick poor were deeply resented by the medical profession, Greer recounts, which alleged that they offered free treatment to people who could afford to pay, even as they provided the medical schools means to teach students, improve diagnostics, and advance careers. Health departments, developed following the Civil War to combat epidemics like cholera and yellow fever, were likewise opposed by the profession when they extended their activities from sanitation efforts to diagnosis and treatment of such diseases, he notes. The president of the New York County Medical Society told members in 1897 that the New York health department was "usurping the duties, rights and privileges of the medical profession" (Greer, 1990, pp. 207–208) when it required reporting and notification of tuberculosis cases and offered treatment. Even the medical schools soon found their pre-Flexner ambulatory medical sites, once so useful in training staff and students, financially and organizationally unattractive.

Ultimately, these socially responsive sites of ambulatory education, the return of which we presently seek, were sacrificed to the educational reforms of the early 20th century, when the number of medical schools declined and the pool of free labor for dispensaries dried up, much to the relief of the medical profession at large. (Greer, 1990, p. 207)

Physicians with a sense of public mission separated from the medical schools to found schools of public health. As private physicians' interests were thus defended against public health, and medical schools relieved of any charge beyond individual

patient care and related education and research, so the advocates of public health were sidelined from mainstream medicine, and were to become "poor cousin" to the latter.

In the present day then, Greer argues, pilot projects in ambulatory site medical education should be given the highest priority. These might include demonstration projects that provide
patient care for communities, as well as educational and research opportunities; outreach clinics that attract primary-care
faculty by affording access to populations for epidemiologic and
health service research; and group practices founded on an academic–ambulatory model with core primary-care faculty and
residents and medical students included as associates to participate and be supervised according to their level of training. Populations in rural areas and inner cities would likely welcome
such academic initiatives, as would many established practices.
Opportunities also exist within the network of federally supported inner-city and rural health centers, Greer points out,
where "practical lessons in health maintenance and disease
prevention, clinical epidemiology, and cross-cultural communication are readily available" (Greer, 1990, pp. 216–217).

In these ways, Greer continues, medicine could

> be learned in a more normative practice environment and experi-
> ence would be gained in setting priorities, allocating time, estab-
> lishing cost-effective approaches to patient management, and ac-
> commodating personal lifestyles. The community-oriented
> functions would include identifying parameters of health mainte-
> nance and disease prevention, establishing methods of measur-
> ing those parameters, developing cross-cultural communication
> with community residents, collaboration with non-M.D. health
> professionals and evaluating cost and outcome. . . . Compare this
> rich educational menu with the paltry fare being served up by
> our current system and you begin to get some insight on how
> wide of the mark medical education is . . . and what meager re-
> gard academic medicine has had for its social responsibilities."
> (Greer, 1990, pp. 216–217)

It was the Rockefeller Foundation, Kerr White explains,
that helped separate public from private mission in medical education. First, it assisted in founding a series of independent

schools of public health early in the century, in this way ensuring that such medically relevant sciences as epidemiology, demography, health statistics, anthropology, sociology, and economics would be safely distanced from the medical schools, and that the new schools' faculties would have little or no subsequent impact on education, research, and practice in mainstream scientific medicine. Second, it promoted establishment in medical schools during the 1950s of separate departments of psychiatry in which psychoanalysis was the sole approach taken to the psychological complexities of medicine. In this way, it helped deprive medical inquiry into these subjects of any substantial experimental base. Taken together, the two initiatives

> relegated psychological and social factors . . . to increasingly isolated, and frequently denigrated, departments of psychiatry and schools of public health. Both were virtually barred from central roles in the evolution of modern medicine, its theories, practices and educational priorities [and] attracted different types of faculty members and students. Their influence over the decades . . . has been modest, indeed, compared to that of the other "fundamental" medical scientists employing the natural sciences and the biomedical model. (White, 1988, pp. 52–53)

Serving the same separation presently, Greer asserts—notwithstanding academic medicine's recent efforts to offer primary-care education, shift training to ambulatory settings, treat underserved populations, and give more curriculum time to "population" and even "prevention" medicine—is the configuration of the modern academic health center.

> [I]n the splendid isolation of their academic medical centers the professionals have become preoccupied with intramurally developed questions . . . different from the concerns of the excluded masses outside their gleaming aluminum and glass fortresses. The outsiders don't understand what the academics are doing, and the academics are frequently unconcerned with what the "masses" are thinking. [A]cademics have become too content in the academic health center. Their modern monasteries are comfortable, contained, supportive institutions dedicated to the care and feeding of the professional establishment. Reaching out, learning to deal with different organizational and human prob-

lems, and becoming involved in the complexities of the larger society threaten loss of control and destabilization. They feel secure in tightly contained hospitals where tasks are neatly divided among well-delineated specialties. . . . Finally, the financial incentives are perverse. Although the blame for this falls primarily on agencies outside the academic community, academic medicine has benefited from the perversities. There is more money in inpatient specialty practice than in community work. (Greer, 1990, p. 211–212)

Curriculum

Vast changes in curriculum content since 1910 have not brought any comparable change in structure. Despite notable efforts to integrate basic and clinical sciences, medical education still counts about 2 years of basic sciences in the same array of disciplines followed by 2 years of clinical medicine. The same division of clinics into general undergraduate and specialized graduate training still obtains and the same faculty often teach medical students and residents concurrently. Preclinical and clinical studies have developed so separately for so long now, in fact, that few shared principles exist.

Only one of the negative consequences of clinical and preclinical studies' separate development and lack of shared principles, in Kerr White's view, is the fact that "huge lengthy textbooks" are now written in both areas "in which everything is recounted in great descriptive detail and supposed to be learned available to recall on demand" (White, 1988, p. 60). Curriculum develops without any heed to balance, connection, integration, and, "worse, there seem to be few effective mechanisms for fundamental review and change. Like the organization of the hospital and health services generally it is a top-down, supply-side approach. . . . [B]alance among the full range of sciences fundamental to medicine's task needs radical rethinking" (White, 1988, p. 61).

For their part, Robert Ebert and Eli Ginzberg see the medical curriculum as having taken a back seat, in terms of faculty interest and emphasis, to graduate medical education over the entire postwar period. Within the 4 years allotted to undergraduate medical education, they contend, preclinical instruction, despite periodic reform efforts, has relied on lectures loaded with technical information, and clinical education, assuming that students will specialize over a minimum of 3 years' postdoctoral clinical training, has been geared to specialty and subspecialty medicine (Ebert & Ginzberg, 1988).

Alarmingly, believe Ebert and Ginzberg, academic health centers have become more, not less, detached from the universities in the postwar period exactly as they became increasingly involved in providing medical services. Physician education grew longer over the same period, as residency or fellowship training became the norm. Three to 7 years of postgraduate instruction became a far more important part of clinical education than the several years of medical school. Faculties grew huge in response to the needs not of medical student teaching but of research, graduate medical education, and patient care. Thus the structure of medical education itself has changed little, in contrast to research and service activities, and continues to reflect the two great divides between preclinical and clinical and undergraduate and graduate instruction. With medical schools now responsible for half or less of physician education in the U.S. and with each half under a separate system of oversight and control, Ebert and Ginzberg declare, a serious discontinuity in the educational experience is apparent. Now, its very structure—4 years of college, 4 years of medical school, 3 to 7 years of graduate work—sharply curtails the adaptive ability of medical education, making it "almost impossible to introduce new subjects into an already overcrowded medical school curriculum, which, in part, reflects redundancies between college science and medical school science as well as between clinical experience in the last two years of medical school and clinical experience during three to seven years of graduate medical education" (Ebert & Ginzberg, 1988, pp. 18–19). A result of such discontinuity, according to Ebert and Ginzberg, is the schools' confusion over mission, whether preparation for specialty practice or general medical education and, if the latter, to what end?

Were the rigid structure changed within and among the three segments of medical education, Ebert and Ginzberg suggest, the time required to train a primary-care physician, or a specialist, could be reduced considerably without sacrificing quality. Oxford and Cambridge students, for example, complete the first year and a half of medical school before receiving the B.A. in physiology.

> For good students, therefore, the problem appears to be more a question of turf than of education. There are numerous examples of successful programs that have bridged the college experience and the first two years of medical school. Many students are fully qualified to enter medical schools at the end of their third year of college, a practice that was widespread before World War II and that has had its emulators in recent decades. (Ebert & Ginzberg, 1988, p. 22)

On the other side too, 4 consecutive years of clinical training—the last 2 undergraduate and the first 2 graduate—interspersed with course work are adequate for preparing the general internist, pediatrician, and family physician. As it is, much of a fourth-year medical student's time is spent in elective courses outside of any coherent educational plan and in securing residency training, note Ebert and Ginzberg. With an opportunity to plan 4 rather than 2 years of clinical experience, clinical faculty could certainly design a more rational curriculum. The argument that students profit by going to different institutions for residency training, they conclude, or that a 6-year integrated program would be unduly restrictive, could be met if selected medical schools were to form consortia to exchange students for parts of their undergraduate or graduate experience (Ebert & Ginzberg, 1988, p. 23).

Internal Authority

Leadership

Medical school leaders must lead or be led into adapting medical education to the sweeping changes underway in health care delivery. Third-party payers—investor-owned entities, insurance conglomerates, labor and consumer groups, municipalities—are all transforming delivery methods, and medical practice is shifting accordingly: from fee-for-service to prepaid plans; from independent diagnosis, treatment, and referral to group norms and protocols and approved specialist lists; from docile patients to shared decisions; from physician dominance to shared authority with nurses, paramedics, and technicians.

Neither the lengthening of medical education over the postwar period nor the ceding of responsibility for graduate medical education to teaching hospitals, residency review committees, and specialty societies has been the result of considered planning, Robert Ebert and Eli Ginzberg charge. In contrast, improving medical education, making it less expensive, even shortening it, will require both planning and leadership.

> At a time when the public, third-party payers, and government are taking far-reaching actions that will force significant changes in medical education, the question is whether the medical educational leadership will lead or be coerced into initiating the many changes that are long overdue. . . . While the reforms that we have recommended involve other constituencies than those directly concerned with medical education, including third-party payers, state and federal governments, the corporate community, and philanthropy, the initiative must come from the leadership of academic medical centers. We hope that the leadership of the AHCs will initiate necessary reforms rather than wait for others to force . . . far less desirable alterations. (Ebert & Ginzberg, 1988, pp. 32–33, 37)

Leadership, suggest Ebert and Ginzberg, must recognize that the physician–gatekeeper approach in managed-care settings is catching hold and that primary-care physicians will increasingly decide and make referrals to specialists. As physician practice changes fundamentally—from fee-for-service to prepaid group practice membership based on salary and risk-sharing; independent diagnosis and treatment to group norms and protocols; discretion in referrals to specialists to approved lists and pressure to minimize referrals; instructing obedient patients to exploring their preferences and making joint decisions; respected professional status to being perceived as a practitioner in a demystified field whose members may be sued when they err—so too must physician education.

If the profession and its academic leaders do not move to adapt education to changing practice, Kerr White adds, then it

will likely be the health care corporations in conjunction with
investor-owned entities, insurance companies, labor unions, hospitals, consumer groups, municipalities, and political jurisdic-
tions that do so (White, 1988).

For the educators to clarify for themselves which changes
are needed, David Greer proposes, a national conference might
be convened by the government and major interested foundations in order to forge consensus concerning both obstacles to
and goals for achieving a more socially responsive medical education system. If a conference of the sort were to address the social organization of medical education, it might recommend

> recomposing public academic medical center governing boards in
> a more community-constituent representative fashion; integrat-
> ing medical schools' educational, research, and service missions
> better, for example by unifying the many separate institutional
> approaches to a medical school, its teaching hospitals, and partic-
> ipating community health care facilities, and by coordinating ac-
> ademic and service functions in the community; modifying the
> mission of publicly sponsored academic health centers to protect
> and restore the health of populations, for example by having a
> center's activities guided by ongoing study of its designated ar-
> ea's health concerns, and by adding social utility to the criteria
> for NIH and other research awards; providing direct federal sup-
> port to graduate medical education, instead of through hospitals
> in the guise of payment for Medicare patient services, so as to
> free community-oriented educators from constraints of hospital
> needs and so accelerate development of community-based medi-
> cal education; redirecting support for medical education from sin-
> gle primary care disciplines to joint ventures involving several
> such disciplines; reallocating research funds from biomedical to
> educational research in order to further the development of prob-
> lem-based, community-oriented medical education and thus to
> empower both education-minded faculty and community-based
> physicians; encouraging collaboration between schools of medi-
> cine and schools of public health—to enrich primary care faculty
> in the former by association with the population-oriented faculty
> of the latter and to draw the latter closer into the mainstream of
> academic medicine—extending even so far as mergers to avoid ex-
> pensive duplication of effort. (Greer, 1990, pp. 222–224)

Governance

Decision-making authority is now highly decentralized in medical schools, notwithstanding the operation of schoolwide governance structures. Heads of key departments and divisions have been greatly empowered by the schools' need for resource flows far exceeding education-derived income and their mounting reliance on revenue generated by faculty research and specialized tertiary care. Yet it is precisely to this organization into semi-autonomous research and practice units that some observers attribute the growing subordination of general professional medical education to more revenue-producing activities.

Without direction from a central body, the Pew Commission attests,

health professional schools either have to guess about strategic directions or, more likely, drift along without an appropriate vision. . . . The problem emerged with large independent revenue streams and academic programs in growing health professional schools that had little or no relationship to the university's undergraduate and graduate programs. Left to their own devices, health professional schools have created bastions of power removed from the central mission of the university. (Pew, 1991, p. 16)

Indeed one of the fundamental preconditions to the host of necessary changes in medical schools that Robert Ebert and Eli Ginzberg propose is "commitment at all levels to a new system of governance of the medical schools . . . more attuned and capable of responding to the changing health care system" (Ebert & Ginzberg, 1988, p. 34). In this view, the artificial separation of undergraduate and graduate clinical education is first of all a governance problem. Medical school clinical faculty members, and the national specialty boards and residency review committees that they dominate, the authors explain, control residency and fellowship training outside medical school and university jurisdiction. As such, each clinical department may set its curriculum for residency and fellowship training by rules established nationally that are independent both of other departments and of medical school deans, and each may compete nationally for the best residents with no obligation to train its own medical school graduates.

Inasmuch as power is highly decentralized in academic health centers, residing as it does with the department and division heads that control most of the funding, the result, in the authors' view, is "a confederation of semiautonomous baronies" in which the primary activity of most faculty lies in research or patient care, not teaching. Any significant reform in medical education must therefore "be closely linked to the reestablishment of a core faculty of relatively small size under the leadership of the dean, both of whom see the educational responsibilities of the medical school as its core mission" (Ebert & Ginzberg, 1988, pp. 32–33). Salaries of a core teaching faculty should be covered via hard money, helping shift decision-making power in appointments and promotions, now based on research or practice plan income, from department and division heads back to the dean and the core teaching faculty "where it once was vested and currently is vested in all other professional schools" (Ebert & Ginzberg, 1988, pp. 32–33).

David Greer suggests similarly that if powerful forces have configured the present system so, then comparable force, applied at the level of central governing authority, will be required to change it.

> Academic medical centers constitute a deeply rooted bureaucracy firmly committed to and amply rewarded by the status quo. Power relationships, territoriality, and material self-interest foster resistance that cannot be effectively countered by superficial cosmetic efforts like yet another curriculum reform. Effective measures are likely to be those directed at governance, financial support, and the social organization of the medical school. (Greer, 1990, pp. 218–219)

Greer, too, attributes the immobility of medical schools to their "organization into fiefdoms—departments, disciplines, basic scientists, specialized clinicians, and clinical scientists among others, which represent different interests and are not hierarchically controlled" (Greer, 1990, p. 219). Medical schools now require resource flows that far exceed income derived directly from education itself, he continues, and so they have come to depend on resources acquired indirectly from research and from specialized tertiary care, much of which generated by individual faculty, not by the institution. In this way education has been subordinated "to the requisites of the ... financial needs of the medical school and, therefore, to policy that is determined by interest groups, both internal and external, rather than [by] educators per se" (Greer, 1990, p. 219).

The play of conflicting values, objectives, power, and money is evident everywhere, Greer contends. Federal support for medical education has decreased, and support for allied academic research and specialty medicine has increased, as reflected in the NIH budget and health service reimbursement practices. Harvard announced its "New Pathway" education program just as its affiliate, Massachusetts General Hospital, accepted a $70 million grant from A. G. Hoechst to create a department of molecular biology. States encourage and subsidize family practice education while they push their medical schools' biomedical base to attract biomedical industry. Greer concludes that given the magnitude of such conflicting forces, it is no wonder that curriculum tinkering alone has had so little impact on recent medical education.

Kerr White likewise sees a pressing need to alter governance arrangements, those, in his view, that keep persons "knowledgeable about the impact of psychological and social factors on health and disease out of critical decision-making processes in medical education and research and unable to influence the greater medical establishment's delineation of its task" (White, 1988, p. 53). Barriers to their inclusion include

banishment of family medicine and even general internal medicine "to minor roles with respect to curriculum time, real estate, patient populations, professional status, pay and other trappings of academic power"; most medical faculties' narrow view of the full spectrum of health problems, "their brief, often transient, exposure to highly selected patient populations ... to rare conditions, [to] the 'sickest' patients and the most complicated diseases ... to a small fraction of society's total medical and health problems"; a tendency of subspecialists "to band together [in] self-serving, national organizations closely allied with their bureaucratic colleagues and political patrons, to whom they often seem to owe greater allegiance than to their own universities, hospitals or health care systems, to say nothing of their patients and the populations their institutions serve." (White, 1988, pp. 54–55)

"The medical profession," White (1988, p. 55) admonishes, "must be the only service or production enterprise extant that organizes itself top-down from the supply-side alone; every other service organization examines the needs and demands of its customers, or the demographics of the population served, and plans bottom-up from a 'market,' demographic or epidemiologic information base."

Information generated by institutional evaluation will play a critical role in more effective decision making, the Pew Commission adds. To date, health professional education has defined and measured neither desired outcomes nor progress toward achieving outcomes very well. Few campuses have learned to evaluate either long-term research and teaching missions or short-term funded programs or classrooms. Most are reluctant to ask more substantive questions of faculty, students, alumni, or clients than the usual ones concerning courses delivered or students per full-time-equivalent faculty. Measures of quality and standards of practice—such as curricular guidelines and national board exam scores—do "little to inform individual faculty members or parts of educational programs about the impact of their contributions toward the goals of the program and the activities of graduates in practice." Outcome evaluation, the Commission concludes, "must become the norm" (Pew, 1991, p. 14).

Faculty

Comprising medical school, teaching hospitals, health professional schools, affiliated community and/or VA hospitals, academic health centers (AHCs) arose in recent times on rich diets of research, related training, and subspecialties funds. Along with specialty boards and residency review committees, they now set the scale and scope of undergraduate as much as graduate medical education. Those worried by the trend have urged the schools to reclaim autonomy, shed large affiliated AHC faculty, and retain smaller more dedicated teaching bodies.

Organizations change when change-relevant behaviors and attitudes are recognized and rewarded, the Pew Commission suggests. The current reward structure in health professions education is based on research performance and on patient care, not, despite the rhetoric, on contributions to education. Even where the latter are recognized, they are rarely measured by objective criteria of the sort applied to research and clinical work. Thus, until "contributions to education are measured and are rewarded appropriately, interest in educational reform will be sporadic at best" (Pew, 1991, pp. 14–15).

Academic medicine, Robert Ebert and Eli Ginzberg explain, giving perspective, was completely reshaped by the infusion of National Institutes of Health (NIH) funds that began in 1948. Both clinical and preclinical faculties then underwent an expansion that ran through the mid-1980s and was directly linked to research, research training, and subspecialties development. The academic health center (AHC)—medical school with one or more teaching hospitals, often one or more other health professional schools, often a VA hospital, and one or more affiliated community hospitals with residency programs—was established by the mid-1960s. No great financial sacrifice was any longer required of researchers who opted for academic careers, given how amply research and research training was being funded by the NIH. At the same time, medical school applications began to rise in quality and quantity as the new Medicare and Medicaid programs promised more support for teaching hospitals than ever. Since the 1960s, AHCs have come to dominate advanced medical care, taking direct or indirect control over most residencies, and inducing community hospital aspirations to subspecialty excellence. With the various specialty boards and residency review committees, the AHCs now set the scale and scope of both medical training and the specialty distribution of physicians.

It has recently become clear, however, that a prior article of faith—that AHCs are an integral part of their universities—is not true, Ebert and Ginzberg point out. The medical schools and the teaching hospitals must recognize in this regard that their respective missions and interests in part diverge, that the former should and the latter should not be integral parts of the university. A medical school, accordingly, should have a much smaller full-time faculty whose clinical members are dedicated primarily to the education of medical students and whose fac-

ulty is paid out of the school and university budget and is
wholly responsible for designing the science and clinical curricula. Clinical faculty might then call on affiliated hospital physicians for assistance as necessary and even contract part-time
teachers with the dean's oversight (Ebert & Ginzberg, 1988).

External Authorities

Major Payers

*In the 1980s, major payers cut vital support to medical schools.
The federal government ended direct support for medical education and cut student-aid programs. Congress reduced Medicare
payments for graduate medical education. The states cut residency support and increased tuition. And schools learned that
neither NIH nor capitation grants could be relied on as before to
support programs. By the late 1980s, medical research no longer
saw rapid growth in government and corporate support. These
trends have continued into the 1990s.*

Until now, the Pew Commission records, "a complex array
of support from states and the federal government, patient care
and research" has given massive support to health profession
schools. Now however, "the economic reality of education and
health care is that there will be fewer new resources made available to the educational enterprise" and "schools faced with
static or declining resource bases from traditional sources will
need to find ways of reallocating their resource base to meet
emerging problems and support new programs" (Pew, 1991, p.
13).

Robert Ebert and Eli Ginzberg (1988) again offer perspective. The federal government has been directly involved in medical education for the entire postwar period, early on building
new urban and rural hospital centers, linking VA hospitals with
medical schools, affording beds and salaries for academic medicine, and sanctioning health insurance as a fringe benefit for
federal workers and dependents. In 1965 Medicare and Medicaid began paying physicians and hospitals directly to treat the
medically indigent and elderly who formerly were served by

charity wards or outpatient departments. For nearly three decades, the federal government has paid teaching hospitals both for hospitalization-physician costs and for the direct and indirect costs of teaching. It has encouraged state-supported medical schools to construct or reconstruct university hospitals for teaching and research, covered unreimbursed patient care costs, and helped teaching hospitals attract philanthropic money via favorable tax laws.

The NIH has likewise funded universities, medical schools, and teaching hospitals, the authors continue, for specialized teaching and research in categories such as cancer and heart disease. From 1950 to 1965, Congress funded NIH at an increase of 18% per annum, believing that more money would mean more cure of dread diseases. That the medical schools and residency programs realigned their clinical and subspecialty divisions accordingly, in order to attract dollars and grants, both reflected and accelerated the trend toward medical specialization.

Expansion of the medical schools was also fueled by a perception in the 1960s of a serious physician shortage, a view bolstered by the trend to specialization and by the geographic maldistribution of physicians. By the mid-1960s Congress passed manpower bills to support construction of new medical schools and expansion of yearly class sizes at existing ones. Medical schools increased from 88 in 1964–1965 to 127 in 1986–1987, and graduates doubled from 7,409 to 15,872 over the same period. Academic medicine welcomed the capitation and additional allowances granted.

In 1980, however, a reversal was signaled when the Graduate Medical Education National Advisory Committee predicted medical graduate surpluses and the federal government began halting direct support for medical education. The medical schools were shocked to find that neither capitation nor NIH grants could be relied on as before. In 1986 Congress reduced Medicare payments for graduate medical education. By the late 1980s, student loan and grant programs were cut. State governments began to reduce residency training support and to increase tuition, often steeply. In biomedical research, rates of increase in federal support started to fall in the early 1990s without corporate funding taking up much of the slack. The major payers in health care—government and corporations—have now begun acting together to contain rising costs by a variety of means, including managed care arrangements, substituting ambulatory for inpatient treatment, reducing average lengths of stay in hospital, and using more nonphysician health professionals.

With grants falling over the past decade, say Ebert and Ginzberg, faculty practice plans have replaced the federal government as the major source, at just under 40%, of medical school revenues in the U.S. Surgical subspecialties have led all departments in the ability to bring in income by these means. Concerns over this new source for funding medical education have risen sharply, however, as plateaus are reached due to increased competition for patients and as clinical faculty find less occasion to focus on education and research activities.

David Greer chides the federal government for "its tentative, ambiguous, often contradictory" support for the schools' weak social commitment (Greer, 1990, pp. 203–204). Government, he charges, gives far more support to laboratory-based biomedical research than to primary-care education. Thus in 1988, the NIH granted $4.7 billion for extramural biomedical research and $63.6 million for primary-care training in family medicine, though general internal medicine, general pediatrics, physician-assistant programs, and general dentistry. Also, though government encourages medical education in ambulatory settings, it channels funds through hospitals, which greatly encumbers spending and site selection. It pays indirect medical education costs for services rendered in hospitals but not in clinics. It professes concern for ethical and sociological considerations but provides little related research and education funding. It skews academic priorities by funding hospital-based, technologically oriented specialists on medical faculties even as it decries their reluctance to expand primary-care programs in ambulatory settings. Government, so easily intimidated by the professional establishment, thus finds itself

constrained by deference to the most conservative elements of the academic community rather than [to] the broader population it purports to serve [such that t]he current medical delivery and educational systems are shaped by the needs of the providers rather than the consumers. . . . [T]he Federal Government has shown little courage or initiative in redressing the balance [despite its] tremendous financial and regulatory leverage. (Greer, 1990, pp. 209–210)

Among medicine's perverse financial arrangements, Kerr White includes the facts that hospital care is far more generously supported by the major payers than ambulatory care; that the current reimbursement system is based on final diagnosis ("diagnosis-related groups," or DRGs) rather than on management and resolution of patients' presenting problems; and that procedural medicine pays much better than cognitive (listening, counseling) medicine.

As long as the pecuniary rewards in medicine ignore such elements as time devoted to listening, observing and explaining, experience and wisdom in dealing with interpersonal, domestic, occupational and social stress[, and] simple ambulatory management based on "wait and see" as a diagnostic or therapeutic maneuver . . . it seems unlikely that a more inclusive theory of health and disease will find widespread acceptance. (White, 1988, p. 56)

Discipline and Profession

Many medical faculty are now as mutually unintelligible even across subdisciplines as their overspecialized colleagues are in other parts of the university. Seeking new knowledge and stronger methodologies, medical scientists too have contracted the common strain of "that's not my field" academic parochialism. Their professional associations have secured demand for subspecialty graduate trainees and fostered narrow subdisciplines, specialist subcultures, and the territoriality of specialty boards. It is an ambience quite antithetical, some observers claim, to the general professional education of physicians.

University departments were created by century's end, the Pew Commission explains, "on the notion that specialized knowledge, which could be advanced through a collection of highly trained technical experts, was the way that the disciplines advanced. . . . One of the great success stories . . . is the legacy that such an organization has created in the biomedical sciences" (Pew, 1991, p. 12).

Nevertheless, the model "must be reexamined in light of the current and future changes in health care [which raise] questions and concerns that require integrative and synthetic approaches across a multitude of disciplines and professions" (Pew, 1991, p. 12). The task, the Commission concludes cryptically, "is to keep all that is valuable within the departmental and disciplinary orientation and simultaneously develop a new model that permits new ways of organizing people, knowledge, research and patient care" (Pew, 1991, p. 13).

Professors' allegiance, the Commission continues, is more strongly bound to the discipline and the department than to the central mission of the university. Work is organized by and rewards passed down through departments. The problem is that both

> academic freedom and the general independence of scholarly life that permits an objective pursuit of knowledge pull the faculty away from the cohesive forces of university mission and definition toward their own individualistic aims as researchers, scholars and clinicians. Coordinated institutional reform will require a greater sense of shared institutional purpose. (Pew, 1991, p. 15)

Because professional boundaries, reinforced by accreditation and licensure processes, also limit interdisciplinary contact, the Commission warns, the result is that

> individual professional curricula tend to be isolated [and] support for integrating portions of different educational programs to meet changing health care needs . . . is even more remote. Obviously, these systems of control are also not likely to encourage the creation of new health professionals who, while needed by the public, might infringe upon the perceived prerogatives of their colleagues and existing health professional groups. (Pew, 1991, pp. 15–16)

Weaknesses in the way physicians are educated, Charles Odegaard argues in turn, stem from the modern university ethos, based on the search for new knowledge, concerns for more accurate methodologies, tendencies to specialization, and the split into the scientist and humanist camps. So, in the present day,

> We tend to learn more and more about less and less, and we dismiss . . . the resulting vast areas of our own ignorance . . . saying, "That's not my field." . . . No matter what one's specialty may be, advanced education in the university has made it easy for each one of us to become an idiot-savant . . . an ignoramus about much and a savant or scientist about little. Despite the advantages that abstraction and specialization have brought to us in many particulars, they also expose us to the risk of failing to recognize and deal with context and interrelationships. The risk of an ever narrower perspective is epidemic in the university. . . . Among the environmental hazards for all those who progress through the university's advanced educational process is then the encouragement of parochialism among the practitioners of the professions and the disciplines. (Odegaard, 1986, pp. 71–72)

Joining the modern research university over the last century, medicine has taken a great step forward in physician effectiveness. But it has also, says Odegaard (1986, p. 102), caused physicians to absorb "generalized attitudes about the two cultures characteristically held by members of their immediate group, including a pejorative attitude toward representatives of the humanistic and social culture and their scholarly endeavors."

Still, corrections have been made, Odegaard notes, and, for nearly three decades now, since the initiation of Medicare and Medicaid in 1966, political scientists, economists, psychologists, sociologists, historians, anthropologists, philosophers, theologians, and even lawyers have become increasingly interested in medicine and affect legislative, administrative, and legal changes that have had direct effects on medicine. At the same time, some physicians have taken an interest in the perspective that these disciplines can bring. Thus humanists and behavioral scientists have been brought onto the faculties of some medical schools and physicians have learned to study the nonbiological aspects of medicine. In studies focused on the doctor–patient relationship alone, for example, a great variety of useful findings have been reported by now. The case for medical ethics in the curriculum has been made as well, framed by awareness of the pervasiveness of moral issues in medicine, and the issues of patient competence, consent and refusal, information withholding, and confidentiality have been explored. To retain the biological base for medicine is not at issue, therefore, Odegaard concludes. It is rather the need to broaden that base to include knowledge about the psychosocial and ethical factors relevant to disease and illness.

Kerr White concurs, urging that the sociology and anthropology of medicine receive attention in two ways:

> The first deals with the traditions, culture and practices of the medical and related professions, their institutions and services, and their relationships with patients and populations from their origins to the present, including comparisons with experiences in the cultures of other countries. The second deals with the impact of constructive and deleterious social and cultural changes on health and disease, with the impact of socioeconomic factors on health and also with the ways in which, for example, traditions and cultural practices mold the ways in which patients express and tolerate pain and disability, label or present their health problems, and respond to interventions from different sources. Although covered sporadically by sociologists and anthropologists working in medical schools, systematic immersion in these bodies of knowledge is not part of every medical student's education; it should be. (White, 1988, p. 72)

David Greer focuses on the need to reduce the proportion of specialists and reinvigorate the primary-care education movement. In recent years, he recognizes, agreement has grown that "a socially responsible medical education system would produce a majority of primary care generalists and a minority of specialists, possibly two-thirds to three-quarters of the former. [Yet] the American system still produces a substantial majority of specialists, and the trend is unfavorable [and] the number of medical school graduates entering primary care is [actually] declining" (Greer, 1990, pp. 212–213).

In this, Greer regrets, turf disputes among the various primary-care disciplines themselves have not helped, often creating more competition than cooperation. With no one emerging as clearly superior, and in view of the many obstacles that already exist to bar their development, mergers have even been proposed. Here, with the health care system moving to reimbursement schemes favorable to primary-care medicine and hospitals facing deep financial problems, the primary-care providers at least have the opportunity to act together to meet social demand. The obstacles, in short,

> have been put in place by the professionals themselves: an elitist, specialist-oriented professional culture; the service need for specialty graduate trainees in teaching hospitals; the territorial imperatives of specialty boards; and the reluctance of academics to venture beyond the protective confines of their monastic medical centers. . . . The time for cooperative professional action is now: dialogue, experimentation, pilot projects, joint faculty development, shared courses and clerkships, and collaborative advocacy are urgently needed. (Greer, 1990, p. 214)

Licensing and Accreditation

Broader physician licensing and medical school accrediting criteria have been urged recently to help correct deficits in physicians' nonmedical sciences knowledge, patient management skills, and personal qualities relevant to practice. Thus the National Board of Medical Examiners has been advised to set standards and better evaluate in the human sciences, in communication and interview skills, and in such qualities as integrity, respect, and compassion. Similar changes have been urged on the boards that license specialists and on the Liaison Committee on Medical Education that accredits schools.

"The traditional model of medical education and practice, based largely on organ specific physical illness, is no longer adequate," Thomas Langfitt argues, introducing the Pew Commission's report (1991, pp. iv–v). "Conversion to the new model is the greatest single challenge faced by the health professional schools." Besides the many "educators and professionals [who] believe there is nothing wrong with the present models," he adds, obstacles to conversion also include established "accreditation and licensure requirements [that] discourage the new practices recommended by the Pew Commission." Thus "deans and faculties contend, with good reason, that they cannot change curricula in their schools toward the new models without the cooperation of credentialing and professional reimbursement organizations" (Pew, 1991, pp. iv–v).

Accreditation and licensure, the Pew report explains, introduced at the turn of the century to raise standards and protect the public, now "often impede change within the health professional schools rather than encourage change" (Pew, 1991, pp. 13–14). Like the schools, and in concert with them, the Commission urges, accrediting and licensing bodies must also "think anew" about goals and the best ways to reach them.

Robert Ebert and Eli Ginzberg object to the irresponsibility of specialty boards and resident review committees; bodies that, with no fiscal responsibility for the programs they oversee, nevertheless prolong and elevate the cost of graduate medical education at just the time that the federal government and other payers have cut support for it by reducing patient care reimbursement. Even facing possible surpluses of physician specialists, the authors protest, the boards and committees continue to require excessive training periods of residents (Ebert & Ginzberg, 1988).

Kerr White, regretting the widespread and widely documented lack of interviewing and communication skills among physicians, urges both the AAMC and constituent medical schools and the National Board of Medical Examiners (NBME) to correct the problem. The latter, he proposes, should include a set of exam problems or questions—using standardized patients or one-way screens and standardized interview rating forms, for example, to establish that interviewing and communication skills are important, and the specialty boards should introduce similar standards and examinations. The professional societies of family medicine, general internal medicine, and general pediatrics should likewise become more involved in promoting interdisciplinary and interdepartmental research in behavioral medicine and in setting research and teaching standards. Altogether,

the National Board of Medical Examiners already asks some questions and the Liaison Committee on Medical Education pays some deference to the field in its reviews. The NBME could ask more questions on the final as well as on the Part I examinations and the Liaison Committees could pursue more rigorous questioning during their visits; they should have a behavioral scientist on each review team. (White, 1988, pp. 72–73)

The NBME should also set standards and evaluate students at graduation with respect to their integrity, respect, and compassion, and the AAMC should encourage medical schools each to do likewise themselves, White concludes.

School Functions

Instruction

Medical schools seldom recruit and retain sufficient numbers of primary-care faculty or provide adequately for their teaching and research needs. Medical students thus rarely encounter professional role models who are able to converse with patients or are willing to try understanding the history and meaning to them of their illness and symptoms. The problem cannot be solved, evidently, except by recruiting and retaining more primary-care faculty members with exemplary biomedical and clinical training and the ability to impart listening, hearing, and observation as well as technical skills to students.

"The old G.P. is not the model," Kerr White declares. Rather, it is "the contemporary primary care physician with exemplary training based on the [expanded] model [who a]part from the skills and sensitivity needed to listen, hear and observe . . . will have the requisite knowledge and skills to cope with at least 90 percent of the ills of her or his patients, and perhaps another 5 percent or more after consultations from subspecialists" (White, 1988, p. 57). Younger medical faculty members at the Wickenburg conference, White (1988, p. 36) notes, argued that physician–patient communication skills "are not picked-up as the student or resident moves along, nor are they part of some nebulous art of medicine [but] can be explicitly taught and learned." These same faculty, he adds, "argued that acquisition of interviewing and communications skills is not only a desirable, but probably the only means, for both appreciating and applying a more inclusive model of health and disease" (White, 1988, pp. 36–37).

In Richard Ebert and Eli Ginzberg's broad view, liberal funding of research and research training over the course of the postwar period has only reinforced preclinical and clinical faculty members' greater interest in research than in medical student instruction.

> the ... preclinical disciplines ... became in the postwar era the source of some of the most exciting advances in molecular and cell biology as well as in immunology [attracting g]raduate students [with] financial support. [Though] some preclinical faculty members remained devoted to the education of medical students ... the criteria used in the recruitment of new faculty ... tended to emphasize research abilities rather than a commitment to teaching, particularly since junior faculty ... were expected to compete for their own research funding ... often used to cover a portion of their salaries. (Ebert & Ginzberg, 1988, p. 14)

The recent enormous size of medical school faculties, even the one-to-one student-faculty ratio that often obtains, might but does not create a tutorial-like environment for educating medical students, write Ebert and Ginzberg. Huge faculties instead reflect the pervasive emphasis on research, graduate medical education, and specialty practice. Tertiary-care hospitals are less and less appropriate sites for the bulk of clinical training as patients are increasingly worked up before admission, diagnosis-related groups (DRGs) have shortened hospital stays, and much treatment is now being conducted in ambulatory settings.

Clinical instruction, Ebert and Ginzberg insist, must include more ambulatory site education, even as identifying, structuring, and supervising these sites and shifting the funds needed to cover costs will be challenging in an increasingly competitive practice environment. The shift "will not come easy" inasmuch as the "principal source of financing for graduate medical education is patient care reimbursement derived from Medicaid and insurance" (p. 29). Thus it will require "considerable goodwill and careful planning by payers and providers to have part of the present funding for graduate medical education transferred from hospitals to ambulatory care sites" (p. 29) Critical to making such changes, in the authors' view, is "a core full-time faculty whose primary function is integrating the collegiate/preclinical science interface [and] planning the clinical curriculum up to the first certification of primary care specialists" (p. 25). Engendering a core faculty of this sort will in turn require "recognition that serious teaching is a difficult and demanding activity and that two lectures a year to a large medical school class do not qualify as serious teaching . . . good teaching must be recognized as a primary activity in its own right—and be appropriately rewarded" (Ebert & Ginzberg, 1988, pp. 25–26). Needed to staff such a core faculty, Kerr White adds, will be

> a critical mass of . . . family physicians, general internists and general pediatricians, augmented by psychiatrists, obstetricians and general surgeons, and supported by behavioral scientists, who provide dedicated training modules, including videotapes, for other faculty and residents initially and then for medical students. There is little point in training the latter, if the former two groups do not provide appropriate role models. This is the sort of 'crash program' that the Federal Government should finance, but it may well take a concerted effort by a consortium of foundations to get things started. (White, 1988, pp. 70–71)

David Greer, too, considers the shift to ambulatory and community site instruction and faculty development long overdue.

> Physicians trained in hospitals will tend to stay in hospitals, where their expensive, high-technology, specialty practices can flourish. Students unexposed to and therefore ignorant of the interesting, challenging human and social problems in their communities cannot be expected to choose careers devoted to community service. Education in tertiary care centers exposes students to a narrow spectrum of diseases, snapshots of the evolution of illness, no perspective on prevention, little psychosocial insight, and the most expensive mode of practice attainable. The current educational system is designed for the benefit of the providers not the consumers, be the latter students or patients. (Greer, 1990, p. 214)

Greer also sees difficulty in the shift. Hospital clinics may not be adequate to the task, he fears, given insufficient capacity and narrow ranges of patients and medical problems, whereas other sites—HMOs, large group or solo practices, public clinics—remain to be seen with respect to organization and reimbursement. Questions also remain about who will pay capital costs for added consulting and examining, conference, and class rooms, how quality will be assured in dispersed and varied settings, and where faculty may be found to teach generalist, community-oriented curricula among the sheltered specialists of the medical centers.

Research

Biologically oriented medical scientists often dismiss the findings of the population-based scientists, even though the latter have long shown that unemployment, poverty, recession, divorce, widowhood, and the like take a heavy toll in human illness. Ignoring the fact that it is not the source of results that matters—clinic, lab, or population—but only whether they issue from an inquiring, skeptical curiosity and remain credible, replicable, and useful, "hard" medical science may thus leave the hidden part of the iceberg of disease, disability, and suffering untouched, mislabeled, or regarded as intractable.

What have the population-based sciences been telling us? Kerr White asks. For almost 50 years, he answers,

> sociologists, anthropologists, demographers, epidemiologists and health statisticians have provided evidence that unemployment, plant closings, recessions, deprivation, separations, widowhood, love and support, promotions, job changes, occupational mobility, divorces and other manifestations of the joys and sorrows that mark the struggle for survival take their tolls in human illness and impairments. But these data are generated by so-called "soft sciences" [while t]hose who work in wet laboratories of medical schools have tended to use the term "hard" science to characterize their own contributions. . . . Surely the issue is not whether the evidence is derived from a wet laboratory, a clinic or hospital or from a population. . . . The issue is whether the information generated is credible, replicable and useful and whether the question or problem is approached with an inquiring, skeptical curiosity . . . the qualities that make the effort scientific and

scholarly. No one branch of science, and no one type of evidence has a monopoly on defining credibility. (White, 1988, pp. 27–28)

Though many agree now that the biomedical model leaves "large components of the submerged part of the iceberg of pain, suffering, disability and disease untouched, mislabeled and often regarded as intractable," White (1988) continues, proponents of the broader model have not succeeded in convincing the medical establishment of its merits. Convincing the latter

> is going to take much more in the way of systematic investigation on a large scale to test the broad applicability of the [broader] model [hence] analytic and experimental studies that include collaboration among scientists working in wet laboratories, in hospitals and clinics and in populations . . . coordinated studies . . . that involve primary care physicians, epidemiologists, anthropologists, sociologists, experimental psychologists, immunologists, geneticists, molecular biologists and pharmacologists. (White, 1988, pp. 48–49)

Such large-scale analytic and experimental research projects are scarce in part, White writes, because they are "not seen as important by government and philanthropic funding agencies, by the academic establishment, by journal editors or, apart from a hardy band of . . . neuroscientists and behavioral scientists, by the armies of orthodox clinical investigators" (White, 1988, p. 49) Thus there is "an urgent need for promising young investigators to receive thorough training in the design, measurement and evaluation methods required to test hypotheses bearing on the more inclusive model of health and disease . . . to ask creative questions derived . . . from the lifeworlds of their patients [and] from a broader exposure to the human condition through biography, history and fiction" (White, 1988, p. 49).

Great effort will be needed as well, White realizes, to convince the public and politicians of the rewards, humanitarian and pecuniary, of studying the psychological and social as much as genetic, nutritional, environmental, and biological factors in health and disease. Nomenclature will be a problem in this.

> In particular there are no traditions of providing social and psychological labels or "diagnoses," in addition to the biological; nor

are there traditions for stating the physician's assessment of the severity of the patient's illness and the patient's functional status at various points in the course of management. Much work has been done in these areas, particularly in the development of the *International Classification of Primary Care*. Acceptance of the [broader] model is likely to be facilitated if we provide a[n] appropriate language with which all the patient's problems and medical interventions during the course of an . . . illness can be properly identified, recorded, and counted. Once the distributions of the components of care are known, and the evidence supports the need, the case can be made effectively to change reimbursement schemes and resource allocation priorities. (White, 1988, pp. 78–79)

Even so, positive examples are not wanting, says White, citing the recent founding at McMaster University health sciences faculty, funded by the province of Ontario, of a "Health Information and Analysis Unit" to serve as an "intelligence" unit "to keep the vice-chancellor, the faculty, students and the public informed about the health status of the population served, changes in its status . . . to monitor major changes in medicine, medical education and health services, new interventions and technology . . . to assess their potential impact on the health sciences centers, other related institutions, the health professions and society" (White, 1988, p. 80).

Selection and Admission

Some observers wonder if a balance in student aptitudes more consistent with needs for primary- as well as specialist-care physicians might not be struck in medical school classes. They suggest altering selection criteria to admit more science-qualified nonscience majors typically drawn to teaching and social work, as well as more women, minorities, and rural residents who may be more inclined to primary care and to various underserved populations. Given the profession's fallen public image, they likewise urge admissions committees to assess more carefully candidates' qualities of integrity, respect, and compassion.

The U.S. is one of the few industrialized nations that does not guarantee access to health care for all citizens, the Pew

Commission notes. Thus millions in the U.S. are without health insurance, and less than half of the population below the poverty line qualifies for Medicaid. Rural areas are underserved. Many Americans die prematurely from preventable causes. The number of elderly adults is rapidly rising. U.S. minorities' rate of population growth is more than twice that of the white majority; by the year 2000, 30% of the population will be either Hispanic or a racial minority. Health care, on the demand side, increasingly will have to meet the particular needs of underserved minorities, needs shaped by distinct cultural, economic, and disease patterns. On the supply side, minorities will become a larger part of the applicant pool and entrants to health professional schools and professions. In short, the Commission declares, "Access to health care will remain an important social issue for years to come" (Pew, 1991, p. 10).

On the supply side, David Greer suggests, a more socially responsive medical education system will result from giving medical schools incentives to experiment with admissions, for example, of applicants from rural areas or with less traditional backgrounds. The latter might include nonscience majors, for example, or science-qualified humanists currently attracted to the ministry or to social work who might also be inclined to the human side of general practice and community medicine (Greer, 1990).

Questions were also raised at the conference, White recalls, concerning the composition of medical school classes.

> Do we really have adequate information about the personal characteristics and interests of different types of physicians, especially about those who would be primary care physicians? Are they different from those who are so successful with the complex techniques of instrumentation? . . . Could we not enlist [psychologists'] help in identifying more specifically the balance of aptitudes and talents we seek in the mix of entering medical students? . . . Medical school admissions committees should know what [the] differences are and strive for a more responsive balance than we seem to have today. . . . [W]hat would happen if we selected a large proportion of the classes from those with undergraduate majors in the humanities and social sciences? The facts are that the average acceptance rate [for the former] is 50.3 per-

cent [and for the latter] 42.3 percent [compared] in the natural
sciences [to] 45.7 percent. . . . And those with backgrounds in the
humanities and social sciences do just as well in medical school
as those with natural science majors. (White, 1988, pp. 64–65)

Admissions committees might also seek to assess candidates'
qualities of integrity, respect, and compassion, White contends,
in view of what has become an obvious problem.

[For a] substantial number of patients . . . apparently we now
have a set of labels which betokens ignorance [and] overt hostil-
ity . . . in such dehumanizing terms as "crocks," "trolls," "go-
mers" (Get Out of My Emergency Room), . . . and much more.
Use of pejorative and demeaning clinical jargon to label those patients with difficult, misunderstood or chronic problems implies
that an anti-scientific mind-set has taken the place of humility,
awe, curiosity and the accompanying motivation required to understand and help. (White, 1988, pp. 43–44)

In any case, White concludes, the medical schools should in
admitting, "accord as much weight to competence in the humanities and the behavioral sciences as to [that in] the natural
sciences"; in instructing, "recognize that physicians, more than
most, require . . . opportunities for full development of both left
and right brain functions, the qualities of integrity, respect and
compassion, and a broad understanding of the evolution of their
profession within the context of man's search for a healthier and
happier society"; in preclinical instruction, give "the behavioral
and population-based sciences . . . equal emphasis with the biological sciences [and present] the scientific method as a way of
thinking about our patients' problems and the population's
problems [throughout] the entire curriculum" (White, 1988, pp.
84–85).

The GPEP Report

Because reference to the 1984 *GPEP Report* (Muller, 1984) runs throughout the present document, a synopsis of its contents, as follows, may prove useful to the reader.

Conclusion 1: Purposes of a General Professional Education (GPE)

1. Shifting Emphases: In GPE, medical faculties should emphasize the acquisition and development of skills, values, and attitudes by students at least to the same extent that they do their acquisition of knowledge. To do this, medical faculties must limit the amount of factual information that students are expected to memorize.

2. Describing Preparation for Residency: The level of knowledge and skills that students must attain to enter graduate medical education should be described more clearly. This will require closer liaison between those responsible for GPE and those responsible for graduate medical education.

3. Adapting to Changes in Health and Health Care: Medical faculties should adapt the GPE of students to changing demographics and the modifications occurring in the health care system. Future practice will be shaped more by these changes and modifications than by the traditional medical care system of the past three decades.

4. Emphasizing Health Promotion and Disease Prevention: Medical GPE should include an emphasis on the physicians' responsibility to work with individual patients and communities to promote health and prevent disease. The goal is to balance

acute illness care GPE by equivalent emphasis on health promotion and disease prevention among groups by teaching concepts of prevention throughout all phases of medical education.

Conclusion 2: Baccalaureate Education

1. Broadening Preparation: College and university faculties should require every student, regardless of major subject or career objective, to achieve a baccalaureate education that encompasses broad study in the natural and the social sciences and the humanities.

2. Modifying Admissions Requirements: In framing criteria for admission to medical school, faculties should require only essential courses. Whenever possible, these should be part of the core courses that all college students must take. Medical school admissions committees' practice of recommending additional courses beyond those required for admission should cease. Some institutions may wish to experiment by not recommending any specific course requirements.

3. Requiring Scholarly Endeavor: College faculties should make the pursuit of scholarly endeavor and the development of effective writing skills integral features of baccalaureate education.

4. Making Selection Decisions: Medical school admissions committees should make final selection decisions using criteria that appraise students' abilities to learn independently, to acquire critical analytical skills, to develop the values and attitudes essential for members of a caring profession, and to contribute to the society of which they are a part. They should use the Medical College Admission Test [MCAT] only to identify students who qualify for consideration for admission.

5. Improving Communication: Communication between medical school and college faculties about the criteria medical faculties use to select students for admission should be improved. Medical schools often fail to inform colleges of the qualities they desire in candidates. College advisors often neither understand nor trust stated selection criteria. Admissions committees often say that they

favor broad preparation but then actually favor candidates with high grades in many science courses.

Conclusion 3: Acquiring Learning Skills

1. Evaluating the Ability to Learn Independently: Medical faculties should adopt evaluation methods to identify: (a) those students who have the ability to learn independently and provide opportunities for their further development of this skill; and (b) those students who lack the intrinsic drive and self-confidence to thrive in an environment that emphasizes learning independently and challenges them to develop this ability.

2. Reducing Scheduled Time: Medical faculties should encourage students to learn independently by setting attainable educational objectives and by providing students with sufficient unscheduled time for the pursuit of those objectives.

3. Reducing Lecture Hours: Medical faculties should examine critically the number of lecture hours they now schedule and consider major reductions in this passive form of learning. In many schools, lectures could be reduced by one third to one half. The time that is made available by reducing lectures should not necessarily be replaced by other scheduled activities.

4. Promoting Independent Learning and Problem Solving: Medical faculties should offer educational experiences that require students to be active, independent learners and problem solvers, rather than passive recipients of information. Some medical schools have developed problem-solving methods of teaching that emphasize information seeking, formulation of hypotheses, critical evaluation of data, and integration–application of new knowledge to the analysis and solution of problems.

5. Using Appropriate Evaluation Methods: In medical schools whose programs emphasize the development of independent learning and problem-solving skills, the evaluation of students' academic performance should be based in large measure on faculty members' subjective judgments of students' analytical skills rather than their ability to recall memorized information.

6. Incorporating Information Sciences: Medical schools should designate an academic unit for institutional leadership

in the application of the information sciences and computer technology to the GPE of physicians and promote their effective use.

Conclusion 4: Clinical Education

1. Defining the Purposes of Clinical Education: Medical faculties should specify the clinical knowledge, skills, values, and attitudes that students should develop and acquire during their GPE.

2. Describing Clinical Settings: Medical faculties should describe the clinical settings appropriate for required clinical clerkships and, in conjunction with deans, department chairmen, and teaching-hospital executives, plan organizational strategies and resource allocations to provide them.

3. Supervising Clinical Clerkships: Those responsible for the clinical education of medical students should have adequate preparation and the necessary time to guide and supervise medical students during their clinical clerkships.

4. Evaluating Clinical Performance: Medical faculties should develop procedures and adopt explicit criteria for the systematic evaluation of students' clinical performance. These evaluations will provide a cumulative record of students' achievements as they progress through their clerkships. Faculty members should share timely evaluations with students: they should reinforce the strengths of their performance, identify any deficiencies, and plan strategies with them for needed improvement.

5. Planning Elective Programs: Medical faculties should encourage their students to concentrate their elective programs on the advancement of the GPE rather than on the pursuit of a residency position.

6. Integrating Educational Programs: Where appropriate throughout the GPE of physicians, basic science and clinical education should be integrated to enhance the learning of key scientific principles and concepts and to promote their application to clinical problem solving.

Conclusion 5: Enhancing Faculty Involvement

1. Designating Educational Responsibility: Medical school deans should identify and designate an interdisciplinary and in-

terdepartmental organization of faculty members to formulate a coherent and comprehensive educational program for medical students and to select the instructional and evaluation methods to be used. Drawing on the faculty resources of all departments, this group should have the responsibility and the authority to plan, implement, and supervise an integrated program of GPE. The educational plan should be subject to oversight and approval by the general faculty. Curriculum committees are rarely able to achieve such a consensus. The attainment of the goals recommended in this report will require the existence of an organizational structure that has academic responsibility and budgetary accountability for the entire medical student program.

2. Providing Budget and Resources: The educational program for medical students should have a defined budget that provides the resources needed for its conduct. Expenditures from this budget should be as distinctly related to the educational program as are other funds restricted to specific purposes, such as research or research training.

3. Establishing a Mentor Relationship: Faculty members should have the time and opportunity to establish a mentor relationship with individual students. The practice of having a large number of faculty members, each of whom spends a relatively short period of time with medical students, should be examined critically and probably abandoned. GPE requires not narrow exposure to specialized interests but a broad, general array of knowledge, skills, values, and attitudes, not a glimpse into a narrow area of medicine but breadth and coherence.

4. Expanding Teaching Capabilities: Medical schools should establish programs to assist members of the faculty to expand their teaching capabilities beyond their specialized fields to encompass as much of the full range of the GPE of students as is possible. Faculty members will require help in developing skills needed to be effective, stimulating, guides and mentors. Faculty development programs are needed for this.

5. Supporting and Counseling Students: Medical faculties should provide support and guidance to enhance the personal development of each medical student. Some students may find the challenge of more independent learning stressful and need support and guidance at the same time that they encounter the

standard pressures and encounters with suffering and death that occur in medical school.

6. Providing Institutional Leadership: The commitment to education of deans and departmental chairmen greatly influences the behavior of faculty members in their institutions and their departments. By their own attitudes and actions, deans and departmental chairmen should elevate the status of the GPE of medical students to assure faculty members that their contributions to this endeavor will receive appropriate recognition. Faculty willingness to devote time and energy to an integrated GPE program will depend on whether or not their contributions are given academic recognition.

Other Important Considerations

1. Equity of Access to a Medical Center: For a decade the proportion of underrepresented minorities has not changed significantly. More effort is needed. Tuition to medical schools has doubled and tripled in recent years and has created difficulties that could become actual barriers for the economically disadvantaged and middle-class families alike.

2. Resources Needed for GPE: Research and patient care raise revenues but take faculty members' time and effort. Faculty's preoccupation with these functions is interfering with their engagement with the GPE of medical students. Administrators need to determine resources required for GPE at their institutions and find apposite funds. Tuition dependence should not lead to enrolling beyond resource capabilities. When appropriations are inadequate to program needs, schools must reduce the number of students or increase dependence on faculty-generated revenue. The latter decreases educational quality. Solving the problem of adequate support for private schools will have to involve both foundations and other private-sector agencies and state and federal governments.

3. Accreditation of Medical Schools: If the U.S. Liaison Committee on Medical Education [LCME] and the Canadian Committee on Accreditation of Canadian Medical Schools [CACMS] were to emphasize that the purposes of GPE are to se-

lect and educate students to be active, independent learners and to prepare them for specialized graduate medical education, the dominance of memorization could be reduced and program changes commensurate with the conclusions and recommendations in this report could be accomplished.

4. Licensure of Physicians: Schools' use of the National Board of Medical Examiners' [NBME] multiple-choice tests to evaluate students' achievement and assess the quality of their programs means that faculties have relinquished evaluating authority and that only a limited range of qualities that graduates should have are evaluated. Were only passing or failing reported for the entire examination, the purpose of evaluation for licensure would continue to be served but faculties would not be able to substitute National Board exams to assess students' achievements in each discipline. Thus the heavy influence of these examinations on medical school programs would be diminished.

5. Graduate Medical Education: Though the Accreditation Council for Graduate Medical Education offers some oversight of accreditation policies and procedures, little thought is given to the effect on GPE of changes made in certification or accreditation requirements. Too, specialty program faculties focus attention on the recruitment and training of residents in their fields even when they are responsible for medical student education. Medical students are often recruited so early that it impairs their GPE as students use electives to compete for residency positions. Discussions are needed both within institutions and among certifying boards, residency review committees, medical specialty societies, and graduate program directors to ensure that students can complete GPE without undue stress.

6. New Topics and Disciplines: Numerous groups want to have special areas emphasized, often in existing courses, in the students' education in order to expose students to topics or disciplines that will make them better physicians and/or to attract them to particular specialties. Considering new topics or disciplines, faculties should assess their potential contribution to GPE, favoring those that enhance students' active independent learning skills as well as provide essential new knowledge.

7. Long-Term Research and Educational Program Evaluation: Program effectiveness should be measured not just in the short term, such as by standardized exams or residency place-

ments of students, but also by longer-term evaluation, for example, of how well its students perform later in their careers. Long-term tracking of graduates as they proceed through their specialized graduate medical education into practice should be programmed into the educational research of each institution. Electronic information management now makes such tracking feasible.

8. Continuing Medical Education: Continuing education will become even more important in the future. Successful GPE programs will produce students who need ready access to continuing education. In this, information management systems will be of greater use than periodic short courses to help practitioners pursue new knowledge. Improvements in GPE will require expanding such resources and directing them at systems and program development commensurate with the needs of physicians educated to be independent life-long learners.

References

Association of American Medical Colleges. (1992). *Medical school admission requirements, 1993–94, United States and Canada*, 43rd ed. Washington, DC: AAMC.

Association of American Medical Colleges. (1993). AAMC policy on the generalist physician. *Academic Medicine, 68,*1–6.

Barzansky, B., Friedmen, C. P., Arnold, L., Davis, W. K., Jonas, H. S., Littlefield, J. H., & Martini, J. M. (1993). A view of medical practice in 2020 and its implications for medical school admission. *Academic Medicine, 68,* 31–34.

Bussigel, M., Barzansky, B., & Grenholm, G. Goal coupling and innovation in medical schools. *Journal of Applied Behavioral Science, 2,* 425–440.

Butler, W. T. (1992). Academic medicine's season of accountability and social responsibility. *Academic Medicine, 67(2),*68–73.

Christiansen, R. G., Johnson, L. P., Boyd, G. E., Koegsell, J. E., & Sutton, K. (1986). A proposal for a combined family practice-internal medicine residency. *Journal of the American Medical Association, 255,* 2628–2630.

Colwill, J. M. (1986). Education for the primary physician: A time for reconsideration? *Journal of the American Medical Association, 255,* 2643–2644.

Ebert, R. H. & Ginzberg, E. (1988). The reform of medical education. *Health Affairs, 7,* (2 Suppl), 5–38.

Eisenberg, L. (1986). Science in medicine: Too much or too little or too limited in scope? In C. Odegaard (Ed.), *Dear doctor: A personal letter to a physician.* Menlo Park, CA: Henry J. Kaiser Family Foundation.

Engel, G. L. (1986). How much longer must medicine's science be bound by a seventeenth century world view? In C. Odegaard

(Ed.), *Dear doctor: A personal letter to a physician*. Menlo Park, CA: Henry J. Kaiser Family Foundation.

Evans, J. R. (1992). The "health of the public" approach to medical education. *Academic Medicine, 67,* 719–23.

Flexner, A. (1960). *Medical education in the United States and Canada.* New York City: The Carnegie Foundation for the Advancement of Teaching. (Original work published 1910)

Fox, D. M. (1975). Social policy and city politics: Tuberculosis reporting in New York, 1889–1900. *Bulletin of the History of Medicine, 49,* 169–95.

Friedman, C., de Bliek, R., Greer, D., Mennin, S., Norman, G., Sheps, C., Swanson, D., & Woodward, C. (1990). Charting the winds of change: Evaluating innovative medical curricula. *Academic Medicine, 65,* 8–14.

Geyman, J. P. (1986). Training primary care physicians for the 21st century. *Journal of the American Medical Association, 225,* 2631–2635.

Greenlick, M. R. (1992). Educating physicians for population-based clinical practice. *Journal of the American Medical Association, 267,* 1645–1648.

Greer, D. S. (1990). Altering the mission of the academic health center: Can medical schools really change? In *Education of physicians to improve access to care for the underserved.* Proceedings of the Second Health Resources and Services Administration (HRSA) Primary Care Conference (co–sponsored by the Robert Wood Johnson Foundation), March 21–23, 1990, Columbia, Md. U. S. Department of Health and Human Services, Public Health Service, HRSA.

Harden, R. M., Sowden, S., & Dunn, W. R. (1984). Educational strategies in curriculum development: The SPICES model. *Medical Education, 18*(4), 284–297.

Hughes, E. C., Thorne, B., DeBaggis, A. M., Gurin, A., & Williams, D. (1973). *Education for the professions of medicine, law, theology, and social welfare. A report prepared for The Carnegie Commission on Higher Education.* New York: McGraw–Hill.

Jonas, J. S., Etzel, S. I., & Barzansky, B. Educational programs in U. S. medical schools. *Journal of the American Medical Association, 268,* 1083–1090.

Kassebaum, D. G., Szenas, P. L., & Ruffin, A. L. (1993). The declining interest of medical school graduates in generalist specialties:

Students' abandonment of earlier inclinations. *Academic Medicine, 68,* 278–280.

Kaufman, A. (Ed.). (1984). *Implementing problem–based medical education: Lessons from successful innovations.* New York: Springer Publishing Co.

Kaufman, A., Mennin, S., Waterman, R., Duban, S., Hansbarger, C., Silverblatt, H., Obenshain, S. S., Kantrowitz, M., Becker, T., Samet, J., & Wiese, W. (1989). The New Mexico experiment: Educational innovation and institutional change. *Academic Medicine, 64*(6 Suppl.), 285–294.

Kaufman, A. (1990). Rurally based education: Confronting social forces underlying ill health. *Academic Medicine, 65*(12 Suppl.),S18–S21.

McWhinney, I. R. (1986). Through clinical methods to a more humanistic medicine. In C. Odegaard (Ed.), *Dear doctor: A personal letter to a physician.* Menlo Park, CA: Henry J. Kaiser Family Foundation.

Muller, S. (chairman), (1984). Physicians for the twenty-first century: Report of the project panel on the general professional education of the physician and college preparation for medicine. *Journal of Medical Education,* (now titled *Academic Medicine*) Nov;59(11 Pt 2).

Murray, J. L., Wartman, S. A., & Swanson, A. G. (1992). A national, interdisciplinary consortium of primary care organizations to promote the education of generalist physicians. *Academic Medicine, 67,* 8–11.

Nigro, M. T., & Lynn, R. J. (n.d.). *Reading in medical education: Sources of innovative ideas* (2nd ed.). Washington, DC: Association of American Medical Colleges/ACME-TRI Project.

Odegaard, C. (Ed.). (1986). *Dear doctor: A personal letter to a physician.* Menlo Park, CA: Henry J. Kaiser Family Foundation.

Pew Health Professions Commission. (1991). *Healthy America: Practitioners for 2005. An agenda for action for U. S. health professional schools.* Durham NC: Pew Health Professions Commission.

Rabinowitz, H. K. (1988). Evaluation of a selective medical school admissions policy to increase the number of family physicians in rural and under-served areas. *New England Journal of Medicine, 319,* 480–86.

Riesman, D. (1961). The academic procession. In A. H. Halsey, J.

Floud, & C. A. Anderson (Eds.), *Education, economy, and society: A reader in the sociology of education.* New York: Free Press.

Schroeder, S. A. (1993). Training an appropriate mix of physicians to meet the nation's needs. *Academic Medicine, 68*(2), 118–122.

Seldin, D. (1981). Presidential address: The boundaries of medicine. *Transcripts of the Association of American Physicians, 94,* 75–84.

Smith, L. H. (1985). Medicine as an art. In R. L. Cecil, *Textbook of medicine.* J. B. Wyngaarden & L. H. Smith, Eds. Philadelphia: W. B. Saunders.

Spaulding, W. B., & Cochran, J. (1991). Revitalizing medical education: McMaster medical school, the early years 1965–1974. Philadelphia: B. C. Decker.

Stephens, G. G. (1986). Reflections of a post–Flexnerian physician. In C. Odegaard (Ed.), *Dear doctor: A personal letter to a physician.* Menlo Park, CA: Henry J. Kaiser Family Foundation.

Strelnick, A. H., Bateman, W. B., Jones, C., Shepherd, S. D., Massed, R. J., Townsend, J. M., Grossman, R., Korin, E., & Schorow, M. (1988). Graduate primary care training: A collaborative alternative for family practice, internal medicine, and pediatrics. *Annals of Internal Medicine, 109,* 324–334.

Tarlov, A. R. (1992). The coming influence of a social sciences perspective on medical education. *Academic Medicine, 67,* 724–731.

U. S. Department of Health and Human Services. (1985). Projection of physician supply in the U. S. ODAM Report 3–85. Washington, DC: USDHHS.

Verby, J. E., Newell, J. P., Andresen, S. A., & Swentko, W. M. (1991). Changing the medical school curriculum to improve patient access to primary care. *Journal of the American Medical Association, 266,* 110–113.

Verby, J. E. (1988). The Minnesota rural physician associate program for medical students. *Journal of Medical Education, 2,* 427–437.

Whitcome, M. E., Cullen, T. J., Hart, G. L., Lishner, D. M., & Rosenblatt, R. A. (1992). Comparing the characteristics of schools that produce high percentages and low percentages of primary care physicians. *Academic Medicine, 67,* 587–591.

White, K. (1988). *The task of medicine.* Menlo Park, CA: Henry J. Kaiser Family Foundation.

Williams, G. (1980). *Western Reserve's experiment in medical education and its outcome.* New York: Oxford University Press.

Winslow, C. E. A. (1920). The untilled fields of public health. *Science, 51,* 23–50.

Index

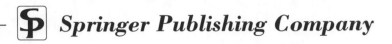

INNOVATION IN MEDICAL EDUCATION
An Evaluation of its Present Status

Zohair M. Nooman, MD, **Henk G. Schmidt,** PhD, and **Esmat S. Ezzat,** MD, Editors

Bringing together the expertise of an international group of 30 medical schools, this new work provides empirical data comparing the effects of innovative versus conventional curricula. The text also examines current issues in problem-based learning, evaluates community-oriented and community-based curricula, presents a methodology for evaluating innovative curricula, and illustrates successful evaluative strategies.

Springer Series on **Medical Education**

INNOVATION IN MEDICAL EDUCATION

An Evaluation of its Present Status

Zohair M. Nooman
Henk G. Schmidt
Esmat S. Ezzat
Editors

Partial Contents:

- Monitoring an Innovation in Medical Education: The McMaster Experience, *C.A. Woodward*
- The Maintenance of Educational Innovations in Medical Schools, *P.A.J. Bouhujs*
- A Study of Ten Innovative Medical Schools: Some Methodological Issues, *R. Richards et al.*
- Perceived Work Load as an Indicator for the Quality of Education, *J. Snellen-Balendong*
- Curriculum Change and Related Evaluation in a Large Established Medical School, *J. Ekholm et al.*

1990   480pp   0-8261-5850-1   hardcover

536 Broadway, New York, NY 10012-3955 • (212) 431-4370 • Fax (212) 941-7842

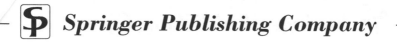
Springer Publishing Company

FOSTERING LEARNING IN SMALL GROUPS
A Practical Guide

Jane Westberg, PhD & **Hilliard Jason,** MD, EdD

Drawing on years of experience, the authors address the questions that educators may have about small group teaching in the health sciences. The first half of the book focuses on practical strategies involved in planning and facilitating learning in small groups. The authors discuss the characteristics of effective groups and emphasize the importance of using a collaborative approach. The second half focuses on planning for and leading small groups that have specific purposes such as providing a forum for discussion and dialogue, teaching communication skills, and helping learners reflect on their patient care experiences, and more. The book's broad orientation and practical emphasis will be useful to all educators in health care.

<u>*Contents:*</u>
- Generic Concepts and Issues
- The Role of Small Groups in Health Professions Education
- Preparing for Leading Small Groups
- Preparing Yourself for Leading Groups
- Leadership Tasks and Strategies During Group Sessions
- Co-leading Small Groups
- Planning for and Leading Groups with Specific Tasks
- Facilitating Discussions and Dialogues
- Doing Problem-Based Learning
- Teaching Communication Skills
- Processing Patient/Client Care and Other Experiences
- Providing Support to Learners

Springer Series on Medical Education
1996   310pp   0-8261-9330-7

536 Broadway, New York, NY 10012-3955 • (212) 431-4370 • Fax (212) 941-7842

Springer Publishing Company

THE POLITICS OF REFORM IN MEDICAL EDUCATION AND HEALTH SERVICES
The Negev Project

Basil Porter, MBBCh, MPH, and
William E. Seidelman, MD

"This is a remarkable book about one of the world's most far-reaching, influential innovations in medical education—the Negev experiment. The authors' analysis of the successes and failures of the experiment is uncompromising in its honesty and self-reflection."

> —From the Foreword by
> **Arthur Kaufman,** MD

Springer Series on **Medical Education**

THE POLITICS OF REFORM IN MEDICAL EDUCATION AND HEALTH SERVICES

The Negev Project

Basil Porter
William E. Seidelman

The authors describe the experimental integration of medical training with the delivery of primary care services in the community.

Contents:
- Health Services in Israel: An Overview
- Primary Care in Israel
- The Negev
- The Negev Project for Improving Primary Care
- The Graduates Program
- Social Work in the Negev Project
- Case Studies: Lessons from the Clinics
- Conclusion: Afterthoughts and Lessons for the Future
- Afterword: What Does It All Mean?

1992   144pp   0-8261-7730-1   hardcover

536 Broadway, New York, NY 10012-3955 • (212) 431-4370 • Fax (212) 941-7842